Why You Are Eating... and How to Stop

Weight Loss Strategies to Overcome Psychological and External Influences on Your Diet

Thomas J Kalloway

derived from various sources. Please consult a licensed professional before attempting any techniques outlined in this book.

By reading this document, the reader agrees that under no circumstances is the author responsible for any losses, direct or indirect, that are incurred as a result of the use of the information contained within this document, including, but not limited to, errors, omissions, or inaccuracies.

Table of Contents

Table of Contents

Cleaning the Plate

I'm fat.

There, I said it. It took me the longest time to admit it to myself. And when I decided it was time I did something about it, I hit a wall that I just couldn't seem to heave my bulk over: calories.

Oh, yeah, I believed in educating myself about weight management, and I found out all about calories, managing them, calculating them, and I eventually ended up hating them. Needless to say, when you hate something, you tend to fail at it. And I began gaining weight, not losing it.

Why was I failing so miserably at losing weight? Surely it was a simple matter of eating less and, therefore, weighing less? It wasn't. You see, I couldn't stop feeling hungry. While I wanted to lose weight, food became my obsession. When I saw it, smelled it, or even heard the sound of cooking, I seemed to turn into a different person. That person was someone I wasn't proud of. That person made me eat and eat and eat. Yet, that person couldn't fill the hole in me. No amount of food could fill up that hole.

I came to a shocking realization: it wasn't the food making me fat. It was my mind. Inside my mind was a person who was unhappy, a person who was conditioned into cleaning a plate, eating what was put before him, and celebrating with food.

My mind was responsible for every pound of extra weight I carried, and it didn't come solely from my food.

Broadening my scope of study into weight loss to include psychology, I finally began to make some progress. My relationship with food, with myself, and with the people in my life changed, and the pounds dropped away.

I am not fat anymore.

I had lost more than just weight, but I was gaining a new life view that was healthier and more beneficial to my continued happiness. Best of all, I could share that life and insights with the people I loved.

It wasn't food that was the problem; it was the things in my life that revolved around food that had been making me put on weight. I had been trapped by my psychology, physiology, social life, mindless habits, and even my own senses had turned against me. Yeah, I used to joke and say I was on a seafood diet—I see food, I must eat it.

Thinking back on those times, I want to weep. If only I had known what I do now back then. My studies had brought me insights I would never have had if not for my deeper understanding of what drove me to feed my pre-programmed needs. I finally realized that I had to change everything, not just what was on my plate. But the results speak for themselves.

Now, I want to share my studies, my revelations about food, and my weight loss strategies with you right here. You can choose not to be fat, just like I did.

My Journey

My name is Thomas J Kalloway and for the last five years I've been studying human psychology and the external factors that influence our diets. I have examined the reasons we're unable to resist eating and, more importantly, how to stop those cold. I've researched the latest proven techniques to stop these outside influences in their tracks and also the methods of regaining as much control over what we eat as humanly possible.

As someone who's struggled with overeating and coming from a food indulging lifestyle, I want to show you that understanding how certain areas of your life are literally controlling what you eat really is the best method for regaining control of your diet and starting a successful weight loss journey. It is about so much more than *what* food you put in your mouth; rather, it is about *why* you put food in your mouth.

Using my methods and understanding the basic tenets of my weight loss revelations will help you make informed and powerful decisions about what you choose to eat and when.

Food will lose its temptation, and you will be able to responsibly plan delicious meals that will help you, not harm you.

I have helped many people on their own weight loss journeys, and I want to help YOU. Overeating is about to become a memory in your past. With my help and skills, you will be able to use all the knowledge and tools to successfully navigate your own weight loss journey. While I will talk a little about counting calories, this is not what real and lasting weight loss is about. It starts with you, not the food you eat!

Instead of giving you recipes, I am going to give you strategies, and those are way more powerful at helping you lose weight.

The methods in this book have shown incredible results, and I want you to join my weight loss revolution right now. People of all genders, ages, races, and sizes have reached their goal weight by using my theories and strategies. This has changed their lives around, and they lost the need to feed the hole in their soul. Instead, I have helped them close up that wound with knowledge, self-care, and love. Scale up your life, not your weight. Here's the first spoonful to digest...

Part 1: The Why of Your Diet

Chapter 1: Physiology and Sensory Influences

If you've ever struggled with being on the heavier side of weight, and perhaps you're struggling with being overweight or obese right now, then you know that losing weight is closely tied to calories. While this isn't the most interesting thing to think about, and calorie counting is no fun at all, it is the very core of effective weight management.

But what about your appetite and ... well, let's face it. Food tastes nice! Eating probably makes you feel good. How can that sense be replaced with a mathematical counting of tasteless calories? I found that when you think of calories as mathematical units, you are not likely to make friends with them. So, let's redefine our relationship with calories.

What Is a Calorie Deficit and Why Do You Need It?

What is a calorie? It's a unit of energy. You eat food, which contains a certain number of energy units, and you live and exercise, which uses up a certain number of these energy units. Great. That's not so hard, is it?

Ok, so now you want to lose weight. How do you go about that? Do you eat less food? Probably a good place to start, but that may not achieve the results you desire. You see, to lose weight you need to put less energy in your body's tank. If you don't use up the energy you eat, then that energy becomes stored in those flabby "battery" packs that take up residence all over your body. Yip, it becomes fat.

So, you need to know how much energy you need to make it through the day. It is not only about how much energy or calories you have in your food. It's about the exchange of energy.

Here's the basic tenet of the law of thermodynamics, which governs the exchange of energy:

Energy is a distinct unit. It can't be unmade. So, you consume a certain amount of energy, and that means it has to go somewhere. It's either used to run your body, like gas in your tank, or it's stored for future use. The same number of energy units (calories) you get out of your food goes into your body. You can't "unconsume" energy once you've taken it in (through eating).

Still with me? Great!

So, according to Andrews (2021), the potential energy we consume from our food is primarily used to work and heat our bodies, and the rest is converted into storage (fat). In colder climates, you would probably need some more calories to burn (like wood in a fire) to keep your body warm, right? When you don't need that extra heat, the wood pile (your body fat) increases.

Therefore, if you want to stop gaining weight, then what you consume needs to match if not be less than what is required for work, heating, and storage. This energy balance is vital for weight loss. If you want to lose weight, then you need to eat fewer calories (energy units) than what you need to work and keep warm. This creates a negative energy balance, which means your body will start to rely on those battery packs you've been adding on with all the supersized meals you've been eating. You will start to convert the fat back into energy that you can use. The result of this is weight loss.

So, how does your body know what you need?

In an ideal world, your body can sense when the tank (your energy levels) is running low. It can either start using battery packs (fat) or it can signal you to take in more energy (hunger, which stimulates the desire to eat). When you are able to only think in terms of energy, you would not "overconsume" calories as this would create a positive energy balance, leading to weight gain.

Why do we eat more than we need then? Surely, if our bodies are telling us that we are stuffed and don't need another bite, we should be listening? Thing is: we don't listen. We are too busy listening to other voices in our heads, and these say things like: I'm not good enough (I'm hungry), I'm not pretty enough (I'm hungry), nobody likes me (I'm hungry), or I'm upset (I'm hungry). These feelings make us believe we are hungry, and so, we eat more than we need, creating a positive energy balance (or fat gain).

Aside from gaining weight through a positive energy balance (when you take in more energy than you need), you will also end up gaining some other things you don't want: plaque buildup in your arteries, cholesterol, insulin resistance, high blood pressure, and an increased risk of cancer. Having more energy intake than you need is not only about gaining weight through energy storage; it's also about damaging your health.

Ok, so you decide to go on a diet, restricting your calories, and you hope you will lose weight. You might do just that, but you find that you still look like a zero instead of becoming a size zero. Your body shape doesn't change. This is demotivating, and you are likely to just start eating a high calorie diet because "clearly it doesn't work for you."

This is where a lack of knowledge is tanking your goals. When you begin with a negative energy balance diet, you need to tell your body where to take energy from; otherwise, it will take the first available "battery" it can find. Sadly, this is just as likely to be your muscles as your flabby butt. You tell your body where to burn energy off through a process of value attribution. What you use will be considered valuable and retained, but what you don't use is storage and can be burned up. So, if you exercise, your body will see your muscles as valuable and build them, taking energy from unuseful areas such as your waist and buttocks where fat is stored.

The short of it is that you need to maintain a calorie deficit (consume less calories than what you can burn through work and heating), but your body keeps telling you that you are hungry and need energy because it's not happy or it's been conditioned to believe it is in a state of energy crisis. Physical activity tells your body that your muscles are necessary, which makes the body protect the muscle tissue and take fat from those wobbly bits you are so unhappy about.

You may want to blame food for your weight gain, but that's "like blaming wars on guns" (Andrews, 2021). Food is not the problem. It's your whole lifestyle and your environment that makes you turn to food. Your mind is hungry; you aren't hungry at all.

If you are an emotional eater, and you tend to want extra calories to feel fuller, then you also need to be aware that your calorie intake can become tipped when your brain convinces you that you are "eating healthily" and "it's okay to have some more because it's a healthy food." So, while a handful of nuts may be healthy, eating a half a cup of nuts three times a day is still overeating and an overconsumption of calories. Your brain can be your enemy.

So, how do you successfully create a negative energy balance or an energy deficit that will result in weight loss? This is the multi-million-dollar question that drives one of the largest industries in business (the health, fitness, and weight management niche).

Your options include:

1. Reducing energy uptake through dieting to decrease your energy levels.
2. Increase physical activity to improve the energy usage levels through physical exercises and a busier lifestyle.
3. Decrease calories and increase energy uptake needs through watching what you eat and how you exercise.

The third one is probably the best option to consider as it tackles the weight problem from more sides than the others. The goal is then to achieve and maintain a negative energy balance, being sure to combine it with physical exercise to help drop pounds. Once you have reached your goal weight, your energy balance can become more normalized as you no longer need to burn fat reserves, you only need to prevent them from forming again. So, if your energy expense matches your daily energy intake, you are on track.

The Hunger Games

While you may consciously understand your decision to lose weight or attain a negative energy balance, the reality is that sometimes you eat before you think. You feel hungry and you act to make that hunger go away.

This hunger is not some little light your brain flicks, telling your body that you are hungry. Instead, it is a series of chemical messengers that travel around, collecting information and reporting back to the home base (your brain) to decide whether you have enough energy (feel sated) or need more (hunger). These chemical messengers are commonly known as hormones.

These hormones can be found in your gut (where food goes into), fatty tissues (your battery packs), and also your pancreas (where insulin is made to control your fat absorption). Some hormones make you feel hungry and others tell you that you've had enough and feel satiated.

Insulin

The chemical transmitter levels, specifically insulin, drop when sugar levels decrease after a meal. This is a natural chemical reaction brought about to tell your body you need energy. This triggers the hunger hormone, ghrelin, to be produced in the stomach.

Ghrelin

This makes your stomach feel empty, and as a response, your brain will create neuropeptide Y.

Neuropeptide Y

This hormone tells your body to eat, increasing your appetite and giving you cravings. The secret to not starting this chemical chain of reactions is then not to let your blood sugar levels drop so low that insulin sends the message to ghrelin, which triggers neuropeptide Y. When you can achieve this blood sugar balance, you will ensure you don't have cravings. This can be hard with a low-calorie diet, but with a positive approach and the skills to manage blood sugar, you can maintain a healthy hormone balance of the body.

Blood sugar or glucose is essential for maintaining a stable emotional level since it's so integrally connected to brain chemistry. Having a mental meltdown can be prevented by a subtle glucose boost before you "lose your mind." Likewise, this is why your brain tells you that you need a sugar fix or some other "comfort food" that will provide the glucose it needs. Of course, there is an emotional component to this too; it's not all chemical and scientific only. But I'll go into more detail on that later.

So, here's the kicker: when you lose weight, it can take up to three years for the hormone balance in your body to adapt to your new body requirements (Truth About Weight, n.d.). While you may successfully lose weight, you still need to consciously manage your consumption versus expenditure to ensure you don't slip back into weight gain due to a hormone imbalance. You may cut back your energy consumption, but if your glucose levels drop too low, your body will make a decision to binge for you. Starvation isn't the answer. So, stop playing hunger games!

There is no quick fix. It is a steady and long-term process of correcting hormone balances and creating healthy habits. This is why popping a pill for weight loss is a short-term solution, and when you stop taking the pills, you pick up the same (if not more) weight.

Your hormones convince your body to eat. They don't ask your conscious permission, and this is why you will find the chocolate bar is halfway into your mouth before your brain catches up and starts yelling, Noooooo, DIET!

Evolution and Diet

Humans have undergone a substantial evolutionary process in terms of our diet. Early evidence hinted at a raw food diet based on the evidence of larger dental structures in early hominids' fossils. Whether this was due to eating raw meat, which is tougher, or predominantly eating harder fibrous vegetables and fruits is unclear. What we eat today has changed greatly from our ancestral past (Luca, Perry & Di Rienzo, 2010).

Certainly, the selection of foods has increased from the foods available to our distant ancestors. Humans have moved from being hunter-gatherers to being pastoral or farming communities. The quality of the foods we eat have also changed substantially, and with this comes the burden of eating hormone-laced factory farmed foods. There is still much debate about the presence of growth hormones in our food sources to increase productivity and how these hormones affect human hormones. It is no stretch to consider that the growth hormones we give to animals to increase their size may end up increasing our size too.

So, from a purely physiological point of view, our modern diet is not setting us up for weight loss success. We have gone from being occasional meat eaters who mostly gathered roots and tubers to being daily carnivores in Western societies. What is the price of this on our health? Meat is acknowledged as being a high calorie food (especially fatty meats) (Web MD, n.d.). While I am not saying you need to change to becoming vegetarian or fruitarian, being conscious about your meat choices is an important step towards better calorie management.

Evolutionary speaking, our ancestors didn't live a life of plenty, and meals were not large. Likely, they traveled during the day, eating nuts, seeds, berries, and roots as they moved about. Eating large meals is then not something our biology was designed to manage. Dieticians will also invariably recommend eating four or more meals a day that are small in size to ensure a steady glucose level (stopping those nasty cravings) and helping your digestion to function optimally.

Yet, somewhere during our evolution, we changed and began eating bigger and bigger meals, loaded with meat and oily foods such as fries and greasy additions. We are eating against our original design. Is it any wonder that we are paying the price with high cholesterol, bad heart health, and stroke rates increasing?

Technology and the Food Industry

The way in which we produce, manufacture, process, and store foods have changed with the advent of the technology age. Demand is high, and as a result, we are pressurizing farmers to grow faster, fatten up animals quicker, and generally create a production line culture in how our food is grown, fed, raised, and slaughtered. There is a price to be paid for this, and being wise about what foods you eat will serve you well in the long run. While GMO (genetically modified organisms) food is cheaper, there is evidence against its consumption as it may be carcinogenic (causing cancers) and have as yet unproven weight gain potential due to the high hormone content in the raising or growing of such foods.

On the processing side of the food industry, fresh foods are not always available depending on where you stay, and as a result, food becomes overprocessed and refined. This is often done to improve flavor, which can mean you will be ingesting additives that are harmful too such as colorants and preservatives.

Instead of treating our bodies with respect, we are turning them into a carnival show for the consumption of culinary creations that are often most unhealthy. Even supposedly fortified foods can be harmful to someone who is insulin sensitive, and we have to wonder why diseases like diabetes and porphyria have increased in prevalence in the past couple of decades. Is it genetic or due to our food choices?

What is apparent is that the food industry is more concerned with meeting demand (and making money) than providing quality sustenance to people. The choice rests with you, and it is up to consumers to educate themselves about what they are putting into their bodies. Organic foods are more naturally grown, and while these are more readily available, they are more costly. Often, foods are altered for cosmetic reasons, such as removing a gene in apples to promote a more glossy skin. The end result is that our scientists are playing around with matters of technology we only have a limited understanding of. We should not be surprised when we pay the price for our ignorance. So, stop shopping with your senses and make wise choices when it comes to your diet and your body.

Senses and Our Choices

If you are anything like me, the thought of Christmas lunch leaves you with a case of serious salivation. Yip, you positively start drooling at the thought of roasts, desserts, crispy potatoes, corn breads, and other wonderful side-dishes. The scent of cooking is so potent that real estate agents use it as a sales technique. Yeah, they spray baking spray in the property they are showing, leaving a subtle hint of "home" to subconsciously make a buyer feel more amenable to buying the property.

We humans are essentially still animals, and we are ruled by our senses. When we smell something delicious, we are moved to want to taste it, touch it, and see it. Cooking shows use this to full advantage with close-up shots of sizzling steaks, roasting golden-brown potatoes, and oozing deserts. While you are reading this, your imagination is even turning against you (and your weight loss goals). You can feel that juicy sensation in your mouth and, pretty soon, you will begin to think you are hungry.

Our senses can provide the biggest challenges to our weight loss goals and diet management aims. Just think of all the times you have gone to the fridge at night, stood there in that halo of light, looking over the shelves for something to eat. Your eyes tell you first, and your stomach responds based on emotional needs. Are you actually hungry when you stand there? No ... but your senses are telling you that you need it. Like sneaky used-car salesmen, they are convincing you need to eat that slice of cake at 1 a.m., when really, you don't.

"Feeding is a multi-sensorial experience" (Luca, Perry & Di Rienzo, 2010). This means our senses are designed to help us find, analyze, and select food. While our senses weren't designed for the modern age with culinary delights, they were designed to help us decide whether a berry was edible or not.

Taste

People, especially adolescents, tend to eat things that taste pleasantly to them. We chase the thrill of a chemical reaction in our mouths that tells us something is sweet, bitter, sour, salty, or umami. If it tastes good, we want to eat it, but if something tastes unpleasant or bland, we don't. This would not be a problem, but often unhealthy food tastes great, which means we crave it due to the taste.

Our tongues lead us into temptation. While adults can reason that something is good for them even if it tastes foul, the same can't always be said for children. If a child is left to make their own food choices, they are unlikely to choose healthy foods due to unpleasant or less delicious tastes. But is this true all over the world?

Depending on your cultural proclivities, you may prefer certain food tastes such as sour or hot and spicy foods. This is something you have acquired from childhood due to your culture. If you are then born into a culture that favors unhealthy food choices, you will develop a taste for those foods. Just think of some world cultures where people happily eat foods soaked in oil or high fat foods. While these foods don't always taste great, the taste has been culturally passed down.

What you enjoy tasting will become a part of your diet. What you don't will be avoided. So, if you are fond of carrots, you will enjoy the taste and eat carrots as part of your diet. Yet, if you don't like broccoli, then you will avoid it, possibly losing out on a valuable nutrient-rich food. Choosing the foods you consume based on taste will not present a well-rounded diet. And if you habitually eat something simply because it tastes good, you are unlikely to be doing your body any favors.

Since taste is a chemical process, it causes the mouth to salivate when a preferred taste is processed. This helps with digestion. Good digestion is essential to the optimal absorption of nutrients, calories, and other useful food components. When food tastes good, it makes us feel more satiated, and thus, we feel emotionally rewarded. This is why when you are feeling emotional, you prefer a nice block of chocolates to a pack of carrots, for instance.

Taste:

- Can help us decide whether something is good for us. When you taste the greasy slick of an unhealthy burger, you can be assured it will be unhealthy for you.
- Is tied to your primitive emotional mechanisms. So, by eating something sweet, you can literally improve your mood. However, the drawback of this is that when you are depressed, you may begin eating candy to feel better every day, causing obesity, which will make you feel more depressed (and eat more sweets, etc.).
- Your taste preferences aren't fixed. What you like today may become unpalatable to you tomorrow. This is often determined by your body's own requirements. If you are low in sodium, you may crave chips.

With taste, we are also greatly manipulated by the sight of something, the smell of it, and the sound of food. Just go watch a movie at the local theater and see what happens when you pass the popcorn counter.

Smell

By far our most potent of senses, smell can help us decide what something will taste like, and whether we will like eating it or not. People can smell over a thousand scents or odors, which can be distinctly classified as spicy, burnt, fruity, floral, resin, and putrid.

When you suffer a blocked nose or upper respiratory infections, you temporarily lose the ability to taste due to being unable to smell. Hence, smell is directly linked to your ability to taste food. It's almost instinctual to smell your plate of food before you start eating.

Driving past a fast food place, just the smell alone can be enough to tempt you off your strict diet and into transgression. Likewise, the sight of your favorite restaurant's signage can be enough to make you suffer cravings. This is why foods are specially composed for photos in cooking shows, on menus, and on billboards and videos of food being prepared always show the process in slow motion to further tempt you.

Essentially, your senses conspire against you. What you see, smell, and hear equates to taste before the food is even in your mouth. The anticipation is enough to drive you into ecstasy with no thought for the consequences of what you have decided to eat. And who is behind all this? The media.

The Media: Pied Piper to Our Senses

Food sells. Simply put, the food industry is probably the top industry out there. Competition is tight, and with many brands competing, the advertiser who can most captivate and energize viewers will have the most sales. There is little consideration for the actual consequence of these sales campaigns beyond pushing a sales point.

We are surrounded by imagery of fries dripping with tomato sauce, burger patties flipping with a sizzle, and chocolate swirling on the end of an egg whisk. This is all so we will rush out and buy a product or consume a certain food group such as promoted by big beef America or even a large chain store fast food group. The resulting diabetes, obesity, and weight management issues that consumers develop is of little concern to these supersized companies.

Sales are driven by our senses. It is increasingly difficult to abstain from eating that ¼ pounder when you see it everywhere, you hear it sizzling on the radio, and you smell it as you drive down the city streets. So, how on earth are you going to make a positive choice to change for a better and healthier lifestyle when the temptation is everywhere?

I am reminded of a conversation I had with a good friend who had chosen to become vegetarian. While she had never been a big meat eater, she still liked chicken, and the sight of finger lickin' good chicken being advertised everywhere was quite an obstacle at first. She quickly realized that buying that juicy family bucket on the way home was more about how it made her feel than how it actually tasted. This meant that she was able to systematically recode her senses, and today, she doesn't feel cravings when she drives past a past favorite shop where she used to buy chicken wings or burgers.

The same can be said for you. It is possible to retrain your brain to not give in to your senses. The first steps are to identify your senses and then to logically think about what you are smelling, seeing, tasting, and hearing. While our senses trigger chemical reactions in our bodies, we can cognitively act on these instead of emotionally reacting.

Food and Seasonal Change

"I'm picking up my winter flab again!" my friend complained, looking moodily at the ever-growing tube she had around her waist. While it was definitely colder, she had gained at least

20 pounds within a month or two. This happened every winter with her, followed by summer starvation diets to fit into a bikini for the beach.

Needless to say, this kind of roller coaster weight management is not safe or healthy for your body. Yet, it repeats each winter, cycling down in summer. So, why do you put on weight in winter? Is it just that it's a cold and depressive season, so you end up eating more bowls of hot and steaming pasta?

The answer lies in our primitive instincts. During the early caveman's time, winter was a time of famine when the herds of animals migrated away and the natural foods they foraged for were harder to obtain under layers of snow. Hence, as a type of life preserving mechanism, as soon as the weather turned cooler, they would start eating more, hoarding food for leaner times when there would be none.

This inheritance is ours today still. We have cravings for carbohydrate-rich foods and dense proteins as soon as fall hits us. We are preparing on some primitive level for the coming lean times, and as a result, we are storing more calories to keep us warm in the winter months. Sadly, those calories are stored as those flabby battery packs I mentioned earlier. Yip, those rolls along your waistline are there as a result of your primitive ancestors. It is survival instinct that drives your jaws during winter. Like an alcoholic who is recovering from their addiction and has to avoid bars, you should avoid places that will tempt your resolve like restaurants and eateries where you know the food is less than healthy. In winter, this need to avoid temptation becomes even more important.

Even today, despite us knowing that there will be food at the corner store tomorrow and the day after and the next couple of months and longer, we still believe instinctively that we should hoard food. It is so programmed into us that our senses conspire to make us eat even more.

Our cultures associate winter with rich and creamy dishes. It's programmed into us. In winter, it's your job to ensure your family and friends can eat rich foods when they visit you. Serve up a salad when it's winter, and you are doomed to family ridicule. Cravings become your culture.

Cravings hit overdrive, and you get the seasonal blues that drive you to enjoy warm drinks and eat large meals. The reward is that warm and full tummy (that you could have done without or with less food on your plate), and so, you overeat. You may be aware you are doing this already, and you comfort your conscience by saying, "oh, it's winter. I'll diet in summer," but how does this affect your body in the long term?

Apart from the obvious damage to your skin with expanding and contracting as you gain and then lose weight repetitively, the damage to your organs is also substantial. Your gut is designed to manage a steady and adequate stream of nutrient-rich foods. It is not meant to cope with an overload as in winter, nor is it supposed to run empty with a starvation diet in summer.

We can conclude that the physiological effects of food present a substantial range of barriers to overcome if you are to manage your weight effectively and long term. The idea is to be able to make informed choices about the foods you consume so these foods won't consume you.

Knowing what foods do, how they present energy, what your body does with that energy, and how these foods influence your mind is part of your weight journey. Now that you have explored the physical, it's time to look at the emotional and mental reasons you have been eating more than you should.

Chapter 2: Psychological Influences

What you think about food is an important aspect of your diet. Weight gain is more complicated than just saying you are an emotional eater. In terms of thinking about food, you need to process information, make decisions after weighing up all the information you have at your disposal, and you may also make subconscious decisions based on information you don't consciously even realize. This is a very complicated process, but if you don't learn to think about food in a meaningful and positive way, you will forever be a slave to your plate.

Let's take a closer look at food and your mental processes, outside factors, how this impacts your ability to reason logically, and how knowledge informs choice.

Mood and Food

The body is run by chemical messengers that tell your different organs what to do. They also tell you what to eat, when, and how much. This is, in essence, how mood controls your food intake.

In the human body, the gonadal hormones of estrogen, progesterone, and testosterone are secreted in the gonads. In women, this is the ovaries and the testes in men. These hormones affect the brain, thinking, and feelings. It is normal for levels of estrogen to dip depending on where the woman is in her monthly cycle, which affects a woman's mood.

The joke about passing chocolate, pancakes, and puppies through the door to your girlfriend when she's on PMS (premenstrual syndrome) is quite accurate then. However, there are complications with women's hormone balances that exceed the normal limits of PMS. Some women struggle with severe depression, which can seriously impact their diet and ability to refrain from overeating. What complicates matters even further is that not all women have an exact clock to their hormones either. While you might mentally prepare for dark and gloomy (and chocolate-filled) days that should arrive about a week before your first bleed, your clock might have other ideas and show up a day or two earlier or later, surprising you and leaving you ill-prepared.

For women, puberty is another stage of extreme hormonal imbalances, which can affect appetite, hunger levels, and emotional eating. Postnatal depression can have a similar impact following birth when female hormones seriously drop following the birthing, which might explain the sudden weight gain after giving birth.

Men also struggle with some hormonal changes that are often age related too. Low levels of testosterone can negatively influence normal eating patterns in a process known as andropause, which like menopause in women can create substantial weight gain. This all impacts negatively on your self-esteem, and to fill the void this creates, you may be tempted to eat excessively in an attempt to self-assure.

The food you eat can also affect your hormonal balances, severely changing your mood. Sometimes your body does this instinctively, but oftentimes, the balance of food to hormones is so out of whack that you need to take conscious action.

Here are a few examples of the interplay between food and hormones (Magill, 2018):

- **Missing Meals**

When you skip out on meals, your blood sugar levels decrease, which can lead to fatigue and overcompensation later. This affects insulin levels, which directly impacts on the hunger hormone system. Instead of eating less, you end up eating more.

- **Selective Dieting**

By reducing the variety of foods in your diet, you will not ingest a suitable range of vitamins, minerals, and amino acids. A deficiency in these will affect hormone production in your body, which in turn, leads to poor mood and anxiety-driven food decisions.

- **Sodium**

While your body requires salt, binging on salty foods might upset your blood pressure, which can, in turn, lead to hormonal imbalances.

- **Comfort Food**

When you are in a poor mood, you may turn to comfort food, which is usually high in calories. This is not healthy as it negatively affects your insulin levels, and it can lead to rapid weight gain, which will induce an even poorer mood or depression. In studies by Prof. Elena Bartkiene (Martinali, 2019), age was found to be a major factor in comfort food cravings. This may be due to a stronger emotional association to high carbohydrate content foods.

- **Taste**

Different tastes tend to elicit different expressions in participants in food studies. Those with depression are noted as having less of a pleasant experience when they taste appetizing tastes like sweet or salty. In the above study by Prof. Bartkiene, those with depression tended to have stronger disapproving expressions to neutral foods or bland tastes.

At this point, you should be realizing that food is about so much more than what is on your plate. You need to eat not only to meet your dietary needs but also your mental needs. Foods are converted into different hormones, and eating the right food can help you maintain healthy hormone balances, limiting cravings. Here's some mental health food advice:

✔ Do eat set meals at regular intervals to maintain effective insulin levels.

✔ Eat less refined sugars and more healthy grains to ensure you maintain consistent energy levels throughout the day.

✔ Include a variety of proteins and different foods to ensure you get enough nutrients to manufacture the full spectrum of hormones your body needs.

✔ Eat omega-rich foods that help in hormone manufacture and in creating stable amino acid chains for hormone production.

✔ Maintain a consistent weight as massive gains or losses can negatively affect the hormones in your body.

✔ Hydrate with water and get enough exercise as this also triggers the production of necessary hormones and neurotransmitters.

Social Media and Our Inadequacies

While your hormones are the internal control mechanisms that influence your food choices, we should look at the external influences too. The biggest of these outside influences is social media. What you see in the world around you has the power to literally and mentally "feed" you.

Being connected with the right kind of people who motivate you can really help you stay on track with your weight loss goals; however, being e-rounded by people who are negative and unsupportive is not healthy for your mental perception of food or of yourself.

Social media breeds low self-esteem. What users fail to realize is that people post their "best side" on social media; this creates a fallacious view that people are perfect (when nobody is). In a society driven by celebrity worship, the temptation emerges to try and be "perfect," which will only lead to a sense of inadequacy when you fail to reach an unrealistic perfection.

Creating a life-long diet that is balanced and works for you is also a lengthy commitment that will not present instant results. Social media promotes crash diets and fads that are not right for you, but you may be tempted into abandoning your own diet to try a quick fix (just because some celebrity has used that fix).

Another side effect of social media is that it creates isolation, and with the warped world view it presents, depression will follow. Depression and isolation will create unhealthy eating habits that are driven by emotions and unbalanced hormones. Sadly, this can become a vicious cycle (Robinson and Smith, n.d.). You may be depressed, and to escape the feeling of isolation and inadequacy, you escape into your screen and social media. Conversely, this triggers further feelings of not being enough or good enough.

While I have helped many people with their weight management perceptions, one of my clients really struggled with this. Melissa was really struggling with weight issues. She really tried to lose weight by eating less, but she couldn't. Melissa was also an avid social media user. She shared selfies on a regular basis, often provoking unkind comments online. This added to her self-confidence challenges. She would look at people she knew who posted selfies showing themselves as skinny and perfect, and she just felt dreadful. Only once Melissa began to limit her social media interactions and began to focus on her own goals did she begin to make real progress in reaching her goal weight.

Social media also has a serious impact on eating disorders. Bulimia and anorexia are serious weight conditions that have life-threatening effects. Obesity is also a major eating disorder, and while you may be struggling with weight, you may not be obese yet. However, social media may convince you otherwise, which could cause you to lose hope and abandon your weight goals, effectively gaining more weight.

According to the National Eating Disorder Association, a link exists between social media like Instagram, Facebook, YouTube, and Twitter and an increase in eating disorders. Unrealistic and unhelpful advice and weight stereotypical imagery can really cause someone who is struggling with their weight to "tip the scale" over to a weight extreme (either gaining or losing too much weight).

Having a healthy body image is essential to achieving the weight that is right for you. When you suffer from an eating disorder, it is usually triggered by some aspect of social media. These triggers could include cyberbullying, unrealistic body images as promoted by cropping of photos, and feelings of exclusion. Since you don't meet some social standard, you are likely to see yourself as being outside of "normal," which will leave you feeling isolated. Depression is a mental condition that thrives on isolation. The result of this isolation, exclusion, cyberbullying, and unrealistic imagery is some deviant behavior in your food perceptions.

The Power of Choice and of Knowledge

When you know better, you do better. Being informed about food and its effects on your body will help you make better decisions about what you eat and what you should avoid eating. However, making poor food choices can also decrease your ability to think clearly and intelligently about food. This doesn't mean that if you eat a chocolate bar you will now become a slow-witted person who only chooses fatty foods. Instead, if you follow a certain long-term diet, you can expect a decrease in intelligence scores. For parents trying to help their children cultivate a healthy eating habit, this is important knowledge to have.

According to Gray (2011), there is scientific evidence of how a poor diet is related to low mental development among children. A diet rich in processed foods such as highly refined starches and carbohydrates can cause a decreased IQ in children. Consuming a diet variety dense in various types of food is best to boost efficient mental development. This doesn't mean that if you pack an apple for your child the day before their math test, they will magically ace it. Instead, this is a long-term commitment to ensure your body has all the components to produce the neurotransmitters and hormones it needs to operate efficiently. There is no quick fix. It starts from day one and should continue for the duration of your life. This is why crash diets don't work.

Eating healthy foods increases your intake of nutrients that the body needs in sufficient doses to function correctly. However, eating a diet rich in carbohydrates, trans fats, and highly processed (and preservative rich) foods will result in poorer cognitive functioning. Eating a healthy, nutrient-rich diet is not optional.

Yet, a reality is that it is cheaper to live off junk food than healthy foods. For uninformed families, money talks, and they may opt for cheaper diet options without being aware of the damage this does to their child's physical, mental, and emotional health. With children being put on "fatty" diets, is it any surprise that large numbers of children worldwide are fat. In the U.S., over 30% of children are not just overweight but also obese (Geng, 2011).

Making a smart food choice today requires knowledge. It's not simply a matter of following some food pyramid you were taught in high school. You need real and accurate knowledge. This means you need to read widely about the foods available in your area and the research being done into foods. You should ask yourself the following questions before considering adding a particular food to your diet:

- ☐ Is it toxin free?
- ☐ Is it organic?
- ☐ Is it produced from natural and unaltered food sources, not factory-farmed or genetically-modified?
- ☐ Is it processed? (And how much if it is processed?)
- ☐ Is it a different food to broaden my diet variety? (Eating more of the same types of food will not help your diet.)

Having considered the psychological influences on your diet choices, it's time to look at the social influences in more detail.

Chapter 3: Social Influences

Oh, I fondly remember holidays in our house when I was a kid. The tables were laden with food. While we weren't exceptionally wealthy, we always celebrated with food. The greasier and richer, the better. A roast was never complete without all the trimmings, and fries were always done in oil. Cakes had triple layers and frosting had extra "something somethings" in. You know, those family recipes that added to the heart and girth in equal measure.

Sadly, this is also where my twisted relationship with food started. I was programmed from as soon as I could walk that eating equated to happiness. Needless to say, I was never a skinny child. If I was unhappy about something, Mom would soothe my feelings with a sugary treat. Our cupboards were always loaded with cookies, fudges, and other treats. It was expected in our family.

When I finally came to realize that what I was pushing into my mouth wasn't doing my body or health any favors, it was a massive shock to my family, who thought I was criticizing them. It took some explaining and some time before they realized that I had simply discovered the error of our habits, and I wasn't pointing fingers at them.

Do you need to eat to celebrate? No. Is it nice to do so? Sure.

However, you don't have to stuff yourself like a Thanksgiving turkey to be happy or to feel nice. Finding and using the principles of moderation and self-control has been life changing to me, and it can be for you too.

I Was Raised That Way: What's On My Plate

While you may never before have stopped to think about what is on your plate, you really should. The food on your plate ... Did you choose it? Or, and it's more likely, you simply eat it because you've always eaten it and was taught to eat it in your home. Your culture, religion, family education, wealth, and knowledge all weigh in on what you were taught to eat as a kid.

It is up to you to question these and make healthier choices.

Convenience Foods

According to Nursekey.com (n.d.), 80% of Americans eat home-cooked food daily, which is healthier (if you have been raised in a healthy eating habit). Shockingly, 43% of adults, according to the source, eat three or more snacks daily. This means you are eating food you don't really need, unless you do so to balance blood sugar levels.

Food choices in the average American home tends to be based on convenience. Takeout is the option of choice for at least two meals per week. This means most people tend to eat food that is not nutritionally dense or balanced at least twice a week. Chances are pretty high that you aren't going to opt for a healthy take-away meal. Most of us stop for a bucket of high-calorie fun or yum at the nearest chain store. Take-aways are usually sodium rich and high in carbohydrates, and they contain trans fats, which all equate to unhealthy food intake.

Cultural Foods

Food is most often part of cultural or religious practices. It helps to foster an identity within the group you were born to or belong to. This is healthy, but what you may eat as part of that culture isn't always. I am reminded of the movie, *My Big Fat Greek Wedding*, where the vegetarian boyfriend is introduced to the Greek parents, who respond with "I'll make lamb" when they hear he doesn't eat meat. While hilarious, this is often a reality. Cultures have certain expectancies, and if you can't or don't want to indulge those expectancies on your plate, it can become a challenge. This is also why many people simply don't even try to eat healthily. They want to honor their culture.

In most cultures, it is also a show of wealth and influence to present a feast whenever you have visitors, which may be often. The impact of this on your health can be extreme. Even a simple habit such as "breaking bread" with friends can have a negative impact on your health and diet. Some of us really struggle with starches and carbohydrates. The bread taken at these cultural times is usually not low glycemic index (GI) loaves either, and probably not simply a slice.

Other customs and cultural foods that could seriously hamper your dieting efforts include:

- Islamic fasting during Ramadan limits eating to the hours of predawn and after sunset. This can negatively affect your diet as you may struggle to digest food that is consumed after dark. Additionally, not eating during the day can also lead to a drop in insulin levels, which can negatively affect your craving levels.
- Following Ramadan, Muslims also have Eid al-Fitr, which is a traditional three-day long feast where delicacies of all kinds are prepared and families visit to share and eat (a lot). While this may only be for a period of three days, it can be enough to break your dieting momentum, causing you to slip back into snacking needlessly.
- Jewish cultural dishes can be as rich, with the latkes served on Hanukkah being just one example. These fried potato pancakes served with cream or applesauce certainly tip scales towards gaining weight. Traditionally, meals are also served with bread, which again, is not the best idea for a healthy diet. Kugel, a rich treat stuffed with cheese and butter, is yet another cultural dish that won't be serving your diet well.

- With Italian foods, "rich" is a given. From breads to pizzas, pastas to filled pies, and wines with each meal, you could easily pack on pounds if this is your cultural heritage.
- While Indian, Malaysian, or Asian foods are often vegetarian, which we would believe to be healthier; however, the large quantities of oil used in the preparations can contribute to an unhealthy food habit. Many of the dishes are fried or served with starchy side dishes like roti, rice, pastas, or naan breads.
- Christian cultural habits with food centers around religious holidays such as Christmas, Easter, birthdays, anniversaries, and other days of saints. The foods consumed could be stuffed buns, pancakes, roasts, breads, and cakes, which again, doesn't do your waistline any favors.

Family Influences

As parents, we all impose our eating beliefs upon our children. If you are a meat lover, you will raise your children to eat meat three times a day. Likewise, if you are vegetarian, you will likely raise your kids to eat vegetarian foods with you. Whether these beliefs are articulated in the family or simply accepted as a given, the influence is long-lasting and potentially damaging. As adults, children often do or eat something because their parents taught them to.

This is not always a bad thing. It's called parenting, and if you are showing healthy eating behavior to your children, you have nothing to be ashamed of. However, if you are not eating healthy at all, then you are loading your child's plate with your own faulty dietary reasoning. Parental beliefs are the invisible sauce that is served on each meal. Become conscious of what you were served as a child and also take ownership of what topping your beliefs are serving your own child.

Health-Conscious Families

If you were raised in a family that is health conscious, you will naturally consider the foods you choose for their nutritional value and dietary content before eating those. As a kid, I grew up in a meat-and-potatoes house, which provided a limited nutritional spectrum to me as I grew up. While I perhaps realized this was not the most healthy of diets to follow, I instinctively chose to eat the same way. My friend, Larry, who grew up in a home where meals were planned according to the food pyramid had a much healthier approach to eating, and he instinctively chose to eat salads, fruits and vegetables, whole grains, and lean meats.

Where you live (or grew up) will also play a huge role in your food selection process. If you hail from a country in the developing world where there is scarcity, you may regularly eat larger portions when available, and you may rely on staple foods like maize and fish, which is what you were raised on. Your culture then contains not just what your parents chose to feed you but also what was available for eating during your childhood.

My father, being from a poorer family than my mother, had the conditioning to "eat what was on his plate" no matter how full that plate was. Mom loved cooking, and as a result, I ended up with huge plates of greasy food that tipped serious starch levels. Your socio-economic status then also plays a huge role in your food choices and your entire thinking about food. Parents give us our food environment and eating modeling. Many parents inadvertently become feeders to their children who eat way more than they require simply because their parents tell them to.

Other habits your family may create could include eating large Sunday lunches, having fish and fries on a Friday or curries on a Monday, or eating dessert after every dinner. While some of these are pretty harmless, you may find that they could encourage negative eating habits such as overstuffing on a Sunday afternoon. Whenever you tie your eating habits to days, it can become a real challenge to a healthy lifestyle.

The number of people you have meals with will also increase your food consumption dramatically. John de Castro, a psychology professor at Georgia University, has found that with the number of people who join your table, your food intake increases by up to 35% for the first person, 47% for the second person, and more for each next person who joins the meal. Eating socially also increases your food consumption, which is why large events like Thanksgiving or Christmas may result in eating until the roast isn't the only stuffed thing at the table (Bayliss, 2014).

Raising Your Children to Slaughter

Would you like to think about feeding your child in terms of fattening them up for slaughter? No? None of us would, but the reality is that by imposing unhealthy eating habits on our children, we are doing just that.

Most of us are taught as children to clean our plate, to not waste food, and to eat all of our veggies. We are told that we can't have cake for breakfast, and we can't eat extra chips, but when we do find ourselves in a position where we can choose for ourselves, we go overboard and eat two slices of cake and French toast for breakfast (because we have decided we can).

What if we rather raise our children with the power of choice? Being given the skills to make informed decisions about what you eat and when you eat can really help you take ownership of your food consumption. Food doesn't partner well with stereotypical thinking. Take the idea of eating three meals a day, for instance. Do we really need to eat three meals? This implies eating because of the time of day instead of eating when we are actually hungry.

Food is there to sustain health and optimal functioning, not to fill you up. Parents who raise their children with the belief they should eat what they are served (as opposed to only eating until they are sated) are setting the table for obesity.

Here's some interesting ideas to help you take control of your eating habits (and reprogram your mind):

- **Eat When You're Hungry**

Only eat when you actually feel hungry, not when your brain tells you that you should be hungry now. Develop a feel for what hunger really feels like. You might decide to take a day to fast, where you ask yourself if the hunger pangs are really physical or mental (and no, a growling tummy doesn't count as your belly screaming for food).

- **Pre-Decide Your Portions**

If you have to eat because you might not have the opportunity later, then decide how much you should eat based on your hunger level, not on what is available. I like the analogy of going to the gas station to fill up my car. If I have space for only a quarter tank, then I will only pump that quarter tank. I'm not going to fill the tank (my stomach) up to overflowing just because the gas (food) is there. Yet, this is precisely what people are doing. They stuff themselves, eating way more than they actually require to keep their engine running. And by now, you know what happens to excess food ... It magically appears in all the curves of your body until you need bigger clothes to accommodate all that extra "gas" you put in your tank.

According to the Centers for Disease Control and Prevention (CDC, n.d.), child obesity has risen to 18.5% overall in the U.S. Increasingly, evidence is pointing towards different cultural groups having a bigger likelihood of child obesity. Hispanic children have a likelihood of 25.8%, and Black children have an obesity rate of 22%, while White children have a 14.1% obesity rate. Contributing factors include socio-economic status and education (when you know about healthy food, you are more likely to encourage healthy eating habits).

Your job as a parent is to raise and parent your child. While putting food on their plate may seem like a good job to you, it may not be cutting it in reality. Your children will carry the food values you serve them the rest of their lives.

What Should You Do As a Parent to Prevent Child Obesity?

- Model Good Eating Habits. When you show your child with your behavior what good eating habits look like, they are more likely to follow in your footsteps.
- Listen when your child tells you they aren't hungry.
- Reward healthy food choices and encourage a diverse diet from a young age.
- Encourage better food preparation and serving ideas to help your child eat foods that may not be as nice tasting but that are healthier for them.
- Teach your child about portion control from a young age and stop telling them to eat all the food on their plate.

Childhood obesity is a serious issue, and you can potentially affect your child in a massively damaging way by the way you raise them. Just think of all the food myths your parents raised you with and how, if you had been raised healthier, you may have never struggled with weight yourself. Reality check: if a child is raised by one obese parent, they have a 50% chance of being obese themselves. When both parents are obese, the risk for childhood obesity jumps to a whopping 80% (University of California San Francisco, 2019).

Fatal Foodie Friendships

Friends are supposed to stick together through thick and thin, but it may be more of the "thick" than you think. Research shows that if your friend is obese, your chances of becoming obese is a staggering 57% (Gwinn, 2019). If you are friends with someone who is slim, your chances of losing weight increases. So, it really is a case of "thick or thin," but it's up to you to choose which. Being friends with someone who is obese increases your risk of gaining weight because you will likely socialize with them and pick up on unhealthy eating habits such as midnight feasts, bags of hidden cookies at work, or getting on a first name basis with the candy store owner. Choose wisely, exercise self-control, and be sure to inspire your friend to lose weight, not fall into their habits and gain weight instead.

Friends can also be excellent supporters with your weight loss goals, but you need to communicate this with them. When you've been struggling with obesity and weight loss for years, it's safe to say food has become your drug of choice. You are an addict. If you are friends with someone who is a recovering alcoholic, you won't force them to go socialize in a bar with you, would you? So, your friends should respect that you are also recovering from your addiction and you can't be expected to go socialize in a dessert bar.

Being friends with a foodie will mean you need to be conscious of each food decision you make. If you do have to hang out in places that you associate with food, then you may want to arrange beforehand with someone to split a meal with you if you know the portion sizes are large. You might also choose to only have a starter and half of a dessert. Don't simply eat whatever appears on your plate, even if your friends are devouring large helpings of food. If the temptation to indulge is too big, you may want to avoid certain friends in food-rich environments if this is proving bad for your weight loss goals.

When food is your challenge, you need to stack the deck in your favor. This may mean forming new healthier friendships and avoiding those foodie friends who always have the richest meals or lunch boxes at work. If you are surrounded by food, it may become difficult to keep your wits about you. So, it's better to start eating mindfully.

To begin eating mindfully, you should take time between bites, really look at your food instead of simply stuffing your mouth, set your cutlery down between bites, and breathe. Your food isn't going to run anywhere, so stop rushing. Give your body a chance to work like it should, and your body will begin to tell you when you really do need to eat.

This concept extends to alcohol consumption too. When your alcohol blood levels increase, you begin to lose self-control and you taste food less, which leads to increased eating to sate your tastebuds. Alcohol is also rich in sugars and carbohydrates, which further adds to the energy balance in your body. When you become inebriated, you are more likely to suffer decreased cognitive functioning, which can negatively affect the decisions you make.

Alcohol also decreases your gut's digestive functioning and limits the nutrients your gut can absorb, which can lead to malnutrition. As a result, your body senses a deficiency and will try to take in more food to make up for the deficiency.

When you ingest alcohol regularly (such as going for daily drinks with friends), your carbohydrate levels increase, but these carbs are easily consumed in your body's processes, actually leaving you with an energy deficit. As a result, you may become hypoglycemic, which means your body will try to compensate by making you eat more (remember the hunger mechanism we discussed in Chapter 2). The result will be weight gain and poor health.

Workplace Woes and Eating Whatever Goes

If you had an idyllic lifestyle where you could sleep in, make a nutritious breakfast, have a healthy lunch presented to you under a beach cabana, and then eat a nourishing dinner around the dining room table with your family, you would probably have a great diet and healthy lifestyle. However, most of us are in the rat race from oversleeping to missing breakfast, wishing lunch would come (only to eat fast food as we cram in more hours behind a desk), and then finally getting takeout on the way home.

Our workplace lifestyles are not only rich sources of tension and stress, but they also provide for a very unhealthy and weight gaining diet. When you delay eating or skip meals, your blood sugar levels drop, causing you to feel hungrier than you are. Snacking on chocolate bars, eating cafeteria snacks, or drinking energy drinks only worsens the problem as your body goes on a sugar roller coaster.

I know you've all been there. You work a long day without even a chance for a cup of coffee, and not feeling like cooking, you end up eating three or four portions from the local fast food joint because you are simply "starving." These work-food-woes are the result of not planning effectively, and the end result is drastic. Studies have found that those who eat junk food at the office tend to consume an average of 107 calories more when compared to those who eat food brought from home. This equates to 535 calories per week and a staggering 2,200 calories per month. This translates to a quarter pound of weight gained each month (SportMedBC, n.d.).

Avoid the workplace gains (of weight, not salary) by planning ahead:

- Keep bottled water with you. Drink at least three (16 ounce) bottles a day.
- Keep healthy snacks on hand such as cut veggies, yogurt, crackers and lean meat slices, and granola bars.
- Cook extra for the next day. Taking healthy leftovers from home for lunch the next day is a great way to save time and still eat healthy.

Accept that eating is a requirement during the day. Even if your diet includes fasting or limited calories, you still need to prepare for when you are hungry. Grabbing a fruit to stave off hunger is better than being unprepared and looting the vending machine in desperation.

Another area where work can really pack on pounds is work lunches or meetings. When you have to attend long meetings and there is food or snacks being catered, the temptation is to overindulge because it's "free." It isn't calorie free, so don't fool yourself. Dinner meetings with colleagues can be as troubling as there is the concept of buying a round (or six) of drinks, and again, since a colleague or the company is paying, you may overdo it, plunging your diet back into the stone age.

The Media and What's Food-Popular

Technology is a truly amazing phenomenon. Most of us have some sort of fitness tracking device such as an Apple Watch or

Fitbit to help us count steps, check heart rates, and even count calories. However, there is also a darker side to technology: social media.

While apps, groups, and online communities are great at helping you stay motivated for weight loss, these same technologies can seriously hamper your efforts to lose weight. Food can be ordered online, and social media loves to run ads on new restaurants to be "checked out," which increases the temptation to eat out, which is statistically associated with weight gain. Instead of eating the meal you had planned according to your weight goals for the day, you end up ordering a carb-rich meal from a new restaurant because it looked so yummy on Facebook or Instagram.

Food trends can help you find new and interesting ways to stay on track with your meal planning, but it can just as easily lead you astray. Seeing images of skinny people online can both motivate and demotivate you. Your focus should be on you during your weight loss journey, yet social media tends to make you look outside, instead of inward.

Food Misinformation and Propaganda

Another downside to social media is the volume of misinformation that it propagates in online posts and fake news channels. In a sense, this borders on food propaganda, as certain sentiments concerning food are pushed upon unaware consumers.

I recall a post I read about some diet where high volumes of fatty food is consumed as fat has higher energy levels, which burn faster, thereby creating weight loss. Clearly, this had just enough truth sprinkled in to tempt the unwary reader, but ended in a faulty reasoning that would cause weight gain, not loss.

While we live in the information age, most consumers are still not fully informed about food choices, healthy diets, nutritional requirements, and the chaos persists as everyone with an internet connection jumps on the bandwagon to shout out their often poorly researched message.

Social influences are some of the most damaging to anyone who wants to eat healthily. It doesn't have to be, but it tends to be. When you communicate clearly with the people you socialize with, you can potentially gain great supporters and encouragers who can help you toe the line of your diet goals; however, if you socialize with people who are set in their ways and expect you to keep socializing like you've always done, you face dietary suicide. From how you were raised, how you are raising your children, and the food friends you keep to the food planning you do for work, you are responsible for what food passes your lips. Don't let your online dictate your waistline.

Make healthy eating, correct information, planning, and responsible family interactions your habit to reach your weight loss goals and keep that weight off.

Chapter 4: Habitual Influences

What is a habit, and what does it have to do with what you eat? Do you eat certain foods on certain days, or do you only eat from fast food joints over the weekend because you "need a break?" These are activities you repeat and they become habits. Other habits may include smoking, drinking, exercising, and a whole range of other activities that you begin to do without even thinking about them.

Some habits are good, but others are really bad for your health. Good habits may be to drink a glass of water before a meal, exercise every morning, and eat slowly. Bad habits may be to only drink coffee, grab food from the corner takeout place (because you're always rushing), and celebrate every occasion with a massive meal.

Your brain uses habits to make life simpler for it. By having a habit in place, it doesn't have to think about every little thing. So, if your habit is to have a donut on Fridays, then you will stop and buy a donut without even thinking. It will be chewed and halfway to your stomach before you remember you're supposed to be on a diet.

Habits can be your saving grace ... or they can be the last nail in your coffin. The decision is up to you.

Habit 101

Forming habits is a process when behavior becomes automatic. It takes around 28 days to break an existing habit or lay the foundation of a new habit. It may then take up to 90 days to formalize that habit until it is unbreakable.

We need habits since they help us become efficient in our lives. Our bodies begin to function on autopilot, not needing to make a decision for every situation, but relying on previous experiences to get us through. This can be a problem when it comes to food though, and a perfectly useful mechanism of habit formation can be turned against us. We may be so used to eating "comfort food" when we are feeling stressed, it becomes a habit. Likewise, we may naturally have the habit of eating a large dinner because that's the way we were raised (a habit formed), so we do this without even thinking or checking calories.

Now, if you have been struggling with weight management issues, the chances are pretty big that you've been indulging in unhealthy habits for more than 90 days, which means you need to systematically break down negative habits that formed and rebuild positive habits that you probably failed to develop.

Habit formation can also help you achieve and maintain healthy behaviors that make achieving and sustaining your weight loss goals easier. When it comes to food, most of our lifestyle habits are there because we have learned to pursue them. We choose to eat large meals on a Sunday afternoon because it's tradition, but really, it's a habit. You may bake or buy a large cake for your birthday because that's how you were raised to celebrate festivities, even though you are living alone and can't possibly eat a whole cake by yourself (but you were also raised to not waste food, so you'll probably eat it all or freeze some for later).

Our families equip us with habits, which we mistakenly call traditions, especially when it comes to food. The minute we associate good feelings with a particular action, such as snacking on Cheetos and ice cream at 3 a.m. when you can't sleep and then feeling better, that action becomes a habit. Next time you wake up and feel like you can't sleep, your brain automatically tells you to go get a bowl of ice cream and Cheetos so you can feel better. The activity has become a default mode your brain reverts to when it doesn't want to think critically of what to do. Habits also become incredibly powerful when you are emotional and not fully in control of yourself such as when you've had a few drinks.

Scientists have broken this habit formation process down to three steps, called a habit loop. The cue is what triggers a habit or action. So, if you are thirsty (the trigger stage), your habit (behavior stage) could be to drink water (a good habit) or coffee (not such a good habit). The reward stage is then to no longer be thirsty. With these three stages being performed subconsciously, you soon have a habit being formed.

Cue	Trigger	Behavior	Reward
A birthday	Need to celebrate	Buying fancy foods and cakes	Feeling spoiled, but also too full and guilty
Eating too much	Feeling guilty at gaining weight	Eating more food because you're overweight already, right?	The conviction that it doesn't matter is soothed with food.
Friday Night Pizzas	Need to relax after work	Eating unhealthy food for taste and convenience	Feeling valued and perhaps even believing in self-care while eating a status symbol (pizza).

Consider the following habit loops. You might see yourself in them!

Habits are formed and maintained by the lifestyle choices we make, and these are based on our family influences, geographical location, and daily routine or time management. By looking at these, we can begin to really evaluate where our habits are coming from, which are healthy, and which we've chosen and which we've had imposed on us through time.

Habit Creators

There are many reasons we create certain habits as opposed to others. Why is it that some children will grow up to be responsible and healthy eaters despite growing up in poverty, while other children will grow up in the same situation and not seem to realize they are overeating? This might even happen in families, where some children are obese and others aren't. What causes or controls the food choices we make and the habits that we create around these? In essence, we are not the only habit creators.

This may seem like a strange concept, but we don't always make our own habits. Sometimes our habits are made by others for us, or we adopt a habit we see. Just think of when your child has a new friend who swears a lot ... pretty soon, they will also begin swearing a lot. The same holds true for food habits. If you are friends with someone who habitually makes bad food choices, you are quite likely to adopt their habits and gain weight with them.

Let's consider the three most powerful predictors of food habit formation. These predictors are also the forces responsible for shaping our food habits and the choices we make without even thinking.

Family

With family, the habit formation starts from your first spoonful of soft food. While you start life out on breastmilk (or formula), you begin to choose foods as soon as the first spoonful starts passing your lips. Oh, your folks may try everything to get you to eat healthy (if you are lucky and blessed with informed parents), and they may do the airplane or the choo-choo sounds as the spoonful of soft mashed pumpkin heads towards your toothless mouth. But you probably keep those rosy lips shut like your life depended on it. Why?

Let's face it, vegetables tend not to be sweet. They have a grainy or fibery texture, and unless you add sugar or salts to them, they can be quite unpalatable when you are still too young to know they are good for you. They are quite bitter tasting, which triggers a primitive defense mechanism in humans. We naturally avoid bitter things when we are very young. Bitter foods make us have an unfavorable reaction. Just look at the faces people pull when they eat something sour. It's instinctive. In nature, sour or bitter foods were usually poisonous, so these were avoided. Hence, veggies get a thumbs down from your primal instincts.

Fruits, on the other hand, are naturally sweet, and they are pleasant to the tongue. Young children easily eat apples, pears, and bananas. Sweet foods trigger a primitive mechanism to help you gain calories to survive in the jungle. Except you aren't in the jungle, and instead of walking long distances with your cavewoman mother as she gathered berries and roots, you are sitting in a rocker or jolly-jumper all day, playing hardly as much as your calorie intake merits.

Our modern lives are so very different from our primitive ones, and while our parents may or may not try their best to present a balanced diet, we are likely to hit up the sweet tastes from an early age. In desperation, some parents simply give their children what they want to eat to keep the peace in the house. Perhaps this is even what their parents' parents did with them when they were children? It now becomes a cyclical phenomenon of poor parenting due to being given what they wanted.

The problem with giving children what they want when it comes to food is the way in which you affect their energy intake. Too much energy, and you trigger weight gain. Our instincts are to eat when food is around (which is all the time in modern life) and to store energy or fats away for when food will be in short supply (which is never, unless you are planning on going on *Survivor*). So, children are fed high-energy sweet diets, and the result of this is a positive energy balance, which leads to weight gain.

Parents may reward children for eating "difficult" foods with other more pleasant foods, which creates an early model for rewarding good behavior with food. A typical example of this is to say, "You can't have your dessert if you don't eat your veggies." While the intention is to motivate children to eat good food, it may create a poor balance of self-control in children. Children raised with this negotiation style will not have effective self-agency or self-control to manage their own diets as adults.

Imagine if your parents never let you eat chocolate after dinner, but your friend's mom offers him a sweet before bed, would you refrain from eating a sweet when you visit him, or would you have several since they are freely available in his home? Being too health conscious with food can also cause problems as the risk of binging becomes increased, like Eve looking at the forbidden fruit. Extreme forms of food regulation can cause difficulties with emotional eating in future.

Children do what they see. This is another primitive survival mechanism, which allowed our ancestors to learn from an early age to walk, speak, and interact by copying their parents. What you eat, your child will eat. If you are modeling excessive behavior such as gluttony, excessive drinking, unhealthy food choices, and other food behaviors that are unhealthy for a sustained and balanced life, your children will copy you. So, if you are prone to getting takeout for dinner, there's hardly any fresh fruits or veggies in your kitchen, and you have bottles and bottles of sodas in your fridge, your children are likely to copy you.

With more and more women working away from home, children are often left at daycare facilities, where the meals may not always be balanced. Traditionally, it was the mother's role to feed the children, yet this is no longer what happens in a large majority of American homes. Fathers may work shorter hours or shifts, making them responsible for feeding the children when mom's not home. If both parents aren't following the same feeding routine, then children may develop poor eating habits. Oftentimes, it is simply easier to give the child what they want and not what they need, resulting in an ever-increasing energy uptake that causes overweight children and obesity in children.

Caregivers, whether familial such as grandparents or employed such as nannies, may not always feed what is appropriate for a child to eat. What seems like an innocent sweet or snack to win over the child's cooperation with doing homework may be the start of major eating disorders.

Lastly, when considering the impact of mothers on children's taste preferences, interesting research (Savage et al., 2007) has found that what the mother eats may become "programed" into the amniotic fluid during the pregnancy. We certainly know that alcohol and drugs get transferred to the unborn child, so why not food too? If the mother is on a diet of high carbs and sugars with less protein and even a deficiency of fibers from natural sources like fruits and vegetables, then the unborn child is literally conditioned in the warm amniotic fluid that it floats in. What the mother eats is the "soup" that her child is growing in. Later, when the child is born, this extends to breastfeeding too, where a poor maternal diet will produce low quality breastmilk. Thus, the child is born and raised with food habits already in place.

Where did you learn to eat the way you currently do? Who taught you to overeat, undereat, drink, or do other harmful things to your body? Where did you first see it? Our family and friends (who are an extension of our family concept) are the ones who teach us from a young age what is expected of food, what is acceptable of food, and how to decide what our relationship with food will be for the rest of our lives—unless we create new food habits.

Location

Where you were born and grew up (or grew fat) could also be a huge contributing factor to the food habits you have acquired. National Geographic's 2011 food chart of what the world eats clearly shows how some differences exist based on geography or location.

The charts indicate that as a whole, the world relies on grain for 45% of its daily calorie intake, while America relies on only 22% of its calories from grain. While the rest of the world gets 20% of its calories from fats and sugars, America gets 37% of its calories from this source. What does this mean? It means quite clearly that the U.S. is a snacking, takeout nation that doesn't get calories from natural sources but rather gets it from processed foods that are high in fats and sugars.

Compare this to a country like Vietnam, where the infrastructure is less developed and people rely on 57% of their daily calories from grain and source only 10% of calories from sugar and fats. Clearly, less developed countries are more inclined to eat unprocessed foods that they home cook, which are lower in calories. However, this is often outweighed by food scarcity and poverty that can lead to malnutrition and other weight issues.

What is the role of your geography then? How does your location influence your diet and calorie count?

You might believe you live in a first world country and lack for nothing, yet your diet may tell a different story. Having all the choices you could want with the foods you habitually consume may not be the very best thing.

In Western countries, people have a range of options available to them, and these all make life easier and tastier (but not always better). Creating opportunities based on the prevalence of quick food places, restaurants, fast food places, and precooked meals means the creation of unhealthy habits.

Living in a more rural area where there are fewer processed foods available could mean a more basic and healthy diet where parents live in more traditional homes, meals are at set times, and food is home cooked. The same holds true for some forms of suburban living. However, when living in cities and in busy areas, the convenience of the corner fast food joint outweighs the long-term goals of healthy eating, and soon, you may have created a bad habit of Pizza Fridays, Freddies' Grill on Saturdays, ready grilled chicken and 'taters on Sunday (not to mention the rest of the week's fast food regulars).

Proximity to these eating places have created a series of unhealthy habits. If you don't believe this to be true, then list the places you regularly eat from (or at). Is there a place you tend to go to at the start of the week? Try this week not to go there and to eat at home instead ... How does that feel? Chances are you automatically take a cab that runs past the restaurants you want (habitually) to support, or you walk past the deli where you buy pastries and rich meats for your lunch meals. Your food is sourced from habits ... What are yours?

How many of these habits are tied to your location? Do you eat the same if you visit out-of-town relatives? How does the presence of these food temptation centers influence your efforts to lose weight? If you want to change the way you think about food, you have to be consciously aware of the potential dangers of the places around where you stay. Like a recovering alcoholic tries not to walk down a street where there are bars, you should avoid the locations where there are unhealthy foods and bad food choices available.

You need to have strategies in place to help you nullify the food habits you have already formed in your area, and you need to work at creating new ones. If that means driving the long way around to get home in the afternoon so you won't have to see the giant M on the building where temptation lives, then that's what you do until temptation no longer knows your name. Other habits you could start forming to break down your bad food choice habits include:

- Not carrying cash or cards with you when you know you need to drive past a fast food joint where you love to grab some food
- Keeping a reminder note in your wallet to warn you not to buy now and cry later (and you could include your current weight and what you want to weigh tomorrow)
- Closing the car windows when you drive past local food places (your nose is a powerful enemy; don't let it betray you)

It's not always about avoidance either. Sometimes the best defense is a good offense, and creating your own more helpful location-based habits can really help you diffuse the patterns of destruction you had previously created. Consider:

- Going to a local fresh produce market where you can buy delicious and visually appealing ingredients that are healthy to eat and make your own meal at home
- Creating a meal routine at home where cooking (which is often what we hate to do) is something we look forward to. You could have a small glass of good quality red wine, listen to some music, and even invite a like-minded friend over to cook and eat dinner with you
- Starting exercising at the park in the afternoon instead of stopping at food places.
- Taking your dog (if you own one) with you when you go out walking as this will probably stop you entering the restaurants and fast food places along the way as dogs are usually not allowed

Habits are insidious since we tend not to see or acknowledge them. The habits we have regarding our geographical area might be even deeper ingrained than those habits we form regarding our relatives and friends. The people we spend time with will, in all likelihood, go with us to areas where we engage in bad habits like going to an all-you-can-eat pub and grill.

Where you live could be as big a poison to your health as smoking or excessive drinking can be. When you start paying attention to where you go, you will begin to see patterns emerge that coincide with your eating habits. Being fat is not just a weight; it can be a place too. Make going to better places a habit and your weight management strategy will improve in leaps and bounds.

Routine

What is your daily routine? All of us have one. It's the habits we do every day. Some of these can be good habits, but others will be not so good, and it is these that can negatively influence your daily routine.

I want to share my daily routine with you before my weight loss when I was still struggling with the thinking that goes into weight and my life, and then I also want to share my routine with you after I changed my thinking around my food issues. Now, I am not sharing these so you can skip to the second one and try to emulate that. It won't work for you, so don't try.

A routine is something YOU create for YOURSELF. You can't live someone else's routine any more than you can live someone else's life. The goal here is to see what habits had formed in my routine and how I managed to identify the bad ones and change them for better ones.

- **Pre-Weight Loss Routine**

Monday mornings started with me dashing out of bed, late as usual. I would grab some coffee, dump a couple of spoons of sugar in it to sweeten a day I was already not looking forward to. Being late, I skipped breakfast, and it was a "duh" to making my own lunch. Still, I was content because I knew a couple of great food places near where I worked. They were in walking distance, but I knew they did deliver, so why waste my precious lunch time walking there and eating in the park or something like that? Plus, I could cram in some more work while I wolfed down some yummy chicken wings and fries in front of my computer.

If I got hungry before lunch, I always kept some chocolate bars in my desk drawer—my own emergency snack stock. I would often have a chocolate bar after lunch as dessert too. I have a sweet tooth, so I didn't see anything wrong with indulging that. Besides, my mom used to hide chocolate bars from me at home, and it was a treat to look for and eat them all.

At the end of the work day, I would join the rush-hour bleed out of the corporate area of the city I lived in, and within minutes, the delicious flavors of hamburgers, pizza, and seafood would fill the air. These were old friends I knew very well, and grabbing my phone, I easily ordered some takeout with instructions to leave it at the drive-thru window for me. The cashier would always ask if I wanted a side of salad, but I just laughed and said, "Heck no! Throw in some apple pie and sauce for me instead. That's all the fruits I need." My parents never bothered with salads. Unless it was potato salad with extra creme fresh. I also had accounts at all these places, so shopping there was really easy.

Back home, I would wonder why my feet were sore since I hadn't walked much at all. But kicking off my shoes, I'd sit before the TV, eating my delicious dinner and dessert. A hot shower would follow and I'd be in bed and asleep for at least a few hours before my insomnia kicked in and I walked the floor of my apartment, looking for distraction, which would usually be snacks.

The other days of the week would follow pretty much the same routine. I was caught in a routine of work-eat-work-eat-sleep-eat-sleep-repeat. While I was gaining weight, I wasn't gaining anything else in my life.

Fast forward a few years, and I created a new routine.

- **My Mindshift Routine**

This wasn't and isn't a fad. It's a routine I created based on my own negative habits to make a schedule that works for me. You will be making your own unique routine by the end of the book, so just be patient.

Now, I wake up at least an hour or 90 minutes before I have to leave for work (I live within a 10-minute commute to work). That time I use in reflecting on my planning for the day. It's now a habit for me to sit at the kitchen table, drinking a cup of herbal tea and update my mobile device with reminders and motivations. I find these are really important to maintain.

Next, I have a bowl of wholesome oats and some berries. On days when I have time, I walk to work. It's only a short distance through the park, and I enjoy the morning scenery. At work, I spend a little time talking to my colleagues, asking about their days, but when they begin to talk about their lunch plans, I politely move away.

At lunch, I head out, back to the park where I buy a veggie hotdog if I forgot to pack lunch, but I usually have some leftovers from last night's dinner or I make a wrap with tuna and lettuce and fresh tomatoes. I take with some tea or freshly squeezed fruit juice in a flask.

Returning to work after lunch, I feel refreshed and can focus better on work. I head out after work, stopping at a local fresh food market where I spend a few minutes just walking between the stalls with their gloriously colored fruits, lean meats, and cheeses. I have come to know a few of the vendors, and having previously told them I was watching my weight, they know what I like and what I can't eat anymore.

It's fun to shop for lean turkey breast, freshly baked whole wheat bread, low fat cheese, and tiny tomatoes for my supper. Tonight, I don't really feel like cooking, but I also know I can't eat from a restaurant or fast food place as the food there isn't my friend.

Armed with the mouthwatering foods I have purchased, I head home. I put on some great music, but as I began warming the skittle where I wanted to make my Cubano style sandwich, the phone rang.

Caller ID: it's Mom.

I would usually have jumped to answer, sharing where I ate, and listening to her regale me with tales of mouth-watering meal plans she had for the coming weekend, and ask if I was coming over.

I love my mom, but I also realized that many of my bad eating habits started with her. Now I am making a habit of not discussing food with her. She didn't understand my food choices at that time, so I had to find ways to not enter into a tempting conversation. I would choose to only answer the phone after I had made my healthy dinner and had eaten a plate that was equal to my body's needs, not my appetite. What I usually ate for one meal, I now easily split into two, saving half the portion for lunch the next day.

It is great! I didn't have to cook so often, and I could do other things in the morning instead of scurrying to work or trying unsuccessfully to make lunch. It took some discipline. After all, I used to love snacking at night. So, now I place my lunch part of my dinner in my lunchbox, making sure to label it as "lunch," and I do constructive things to keep my attention off food.

I have developed some great hobbies now. While I had always wanted to learn how to dance, my own bulk had kept me from it. Now, I go to a local dance school where I have learned the cha-cha, rumba, and I am even mastering the quickstep. It's not easy, but it's a huge amount of fun. Best of all, when I get home, I am really exhausted. My back aches, my feet burn, but my smile is always there … and … I sleep like a log.

As you can well imagine, this routine didn't start in its final form. I had to make some changes gradually. Others I could manage in a few days. Oh, and I slipped back into bad routines a few times, but keeping a journal as part of my recovery process has helped a lot. I really look at my habits. I track my routines, not my weight. Yes, I do weigh myself sometimes, but my focus is not on pounds; it's on my day and how I feel.

What would happen if you tracked your habits and held yourself accountable for them each day? Here's some quick tips to help you start the thinking process around your daily food habits:

- **Think about what you buy**: Your weight doesn't start in your mouth, it starts on the shelf. What you buy is what you will eat, so think about what you are buying.
- **Don't skip breakfast**: It's where your blood sugar gets its boost for the day, and having a healthy breakfast will cut your cravings in half.
- **Meals have power**: Your food speaks to you. I'm not talking about the fatty groans of that quarter pounder extra-large burger you're about to devour. Food speaks in color, flavors, fragrances, and textures. Make it a routine to plan, cook, and eat your food with visual and olfactory pleasure.
- **Ditch the baddies**: Yip, you guessed it. You need to ditch the salt, fat, and sugar that you've been conditioned into believing gives flavor to food. It doesn't. **Make it your habit to smell your food** (before, during, and after the cooking). Fat doesn't smell nice. Salt doesn't smell nice. And sugar, even when melting, doesn't smell as nice as you think. You may argue and say they do, but you are thinking of the finished meals you have been loading up on. It's been your habit to believe they are yummy. I'm talking about raw foods here. When last did you smell "nice" raw fat from a steak?
- **Try new things**: When your habit has been to eat large and to eat heavy foods, it's time to try new things. By eating new and different foods, you won't get bored so quickly, and you will habitually begin to think about

food in a different way, not in terms of that fake fullness it gives you.

At the end of the day, you are the main creator of your habits. You can choose to sustain habits you were taught as a child, or you can decide to change things up for a healthier and happier you. To do this, you need habit awareness. You can only fix what you acknowledge. Look at the people, places, and routines that have made your habits. Question these, evaluate your needs, and make new habits.

It's time to get active, to take action, and to conquer your food challenges. It's time for Part 2 as you take back your food habits and create your own and healthy life.

Part 2: The How-to Guide of Combating Bad Diet Habits

Chapter 5: How to Combat Physiological and Sensory Influences

As we have already learned, your body is designed to ingest food, convert this to energy, which is either used or stored. If you ingest too much energy rich foods, you will have an energy surplus, which is stored as fatty tissue that you can later burn to produce energy when you need it. The trick is you never need that extra fatty tissue. You are surrounded by food all day long, and there is no need to cut back your intake of food to force your body to burn through the fatty tissue. Instead, you eat more and more, creating an ever-increasing store of fatty tissue.

What you eat also leads to your body's ability to store food and excrete what you don't need. This is influenced by your salt and sugar intake, which can negatively affect the hormones in your body.

While you may mentally understand these processes, your biological makeup is gearing you towards failure. This is because your senses—sight, smell, taste, and touch—are all there to help you process the allure of food. You see juicy steaks, you smell rich gravy, and you taste the fragrance of freshly baked pies before you even scoop up the first spoonful.

So, how do you then combat the challenge of your own physiology? This chapter is the start of your recovery process. You've been on the receiving end of the food war, and now it's time to gather your armies and prepare for winning!

The Power of Knowing Why You Eat What You Do

Knowledge is power, and the more you know about why you eat what you do, the better prepared you will be for changing your habits and routines when it comes to food and your overall lifestyle. So, let's reflect quickly on why you eat food that isn't good for your weight management decisions.

What is your food payoff?

By knowing what your food payoff is, you are better able to counter the lure. Your payoff isn't to not be hungry. It could be to not feel lonely, to feel rewarded, to have company, to spoil yourself, to comfort yourself after a tough day, to fit in with friends, or to pass the time.

Know what your reward is, then you can set your own terms. Find out what feeling your food soothes and begin to consider other ways that don't involve food to achieve that goal.

What are your food finders?

When you go fishing, you can sit and wait patiently while you hope a fish grabs the line, you can throw out some bait and hope the fish come closer for a feast, or you can invest in a fish finder device that tells you where the fish are at.

The same holds true for marketers of food. They can patiently wait and hope someone is hungry and happens to stop by their shop or restaurant and buys their food, they can hand out some samples or advertise, or they can use a customer locator (like the fish finder) to tell them where most people are.

This is how restaurants end up in busy places, hotdog vendors know to stand outside office buildings, and fast food places know how to leave the kitchen window open so pedestrians and motorists can smell what's cookin'.

Like a fisherman might throw out fish bait to draw in a catch, the food industry knows how to lure in the "hungry" masses. They appeal to your senses. Knowing which senses you are most partial to can help you prepare your offense.

Do you like to smell food? If you do, then the waft of fresh bread or deep-fried foods will probably have you drooling. Perhaps you love seeing food? Do you have recurring visions if you see adverts on TV with rounds of gherkins gently landing with a wiggle on juicy patties and a brown seed bun? What you see can make you fall face first into your plate.

Maybe you see things in different ways, and the artful arrangement of foods on a plate can inspire you to dive into a restaurant meal.

What is your "trigger?"

Your appetite and hormonal processes will determine why you want to eat something. Your cravings are the result of your "trigger" being activated. By feeling hungry, you know you are about to set off your appetite "trigger!" Find out what sets off your desire to eat. Is it when you are lonely or sad? Perhaps it's when you are angry, and maybe it's when you are happy. Your "trigger" could be set off when you feel sad or overwhelmed and by feeling an overwhelming need to eat. Find your "trigger" and you will be able to control your appetite (and habits) better.

Strategies to Conquer Your Senses

Your senses are the systems that allow you to process information and they operate as gateways to the world beyond your skin. Any system can be changed or rewired though. All it takes is time and strategies. Let's look at different ways to control and minimize harmful influences your senses could have on your food choices; instead, you can choose to find useful ways to explore your senses and your food.

Our Eyes

We see food first. Our eyes focus on what our brain has been programmed with and we focus on food we've had pleasurable past experiences with. This is the simple strategy supermarkets use by placing chocolate bars and chips near the checkout counter. Kids see, they grab, and mommies and daddies have to pay. This is perhaps where it begins. As a child, you were likely also rewarded for seeing foods you wanted by your parents who bought you sweets so you wouldn't put up a fuss if they told you no.

So, how do you counter this? You can't go through life blindfolded.

The mere sight of golden crispy chicken skin or deep-fried lobsters will speak to you as soon as you see them. Even looking away as soon as you have seen temptation will not really help. The image is in your mind, and your primitive side kicks in. The best is not to try and unsee it but rather to avoid seeing it in the first place.

Strategy to Counter Sight Cravings

This means you shouldn't go down the aisles in your supermarket where temptation lives. Stay away from the butchery where rotisserie chickens are turning in the ninth circle of hell or you and your weight management plans will soon be there too. Don't walk down the aisle where the

86

biscuits are and avoid the brightly colored candies and chocolates lane too. Try to pay for your groceries at the self-service counter or the express counter so you don't have to wait and be tempted by those few minutes where the treats are cleverly displayed near the checkout area.

Devise strategies to stop your eyes from wandering. If the lines are long at the grocery store or local deli, then rather browse your mobile, catch up on some emails, or look through the health-wise recipe apps.

Smell

Your next most powerful sense is our sense of smell. It can be so intense that we can actually taste the smell. Another feature of smell is that it often triggers an olfactory reaction, causing our association of certain places, people, or memories that are connected to a particular smell.

So, when you are going bonkers after the smell of fresh bread and deli meats pan fried to sniffing and heavenly perfection, you are not only remembering a smell, but you are also remembering the memories that came with that smell. Thus, if you have fond memories associated with large family meals with a feast of foods, you will have a memory of the happiness those events brought.

Smelling an association of a past memory is loaded with the scent of food and can cause you to eat because of the fond memories you are made to recall due to smell. The nerve cells at the roof of the nasal passages are connected to the olfactory bulb in the frontal lobe of the brain where memories are stored.

Strategy for Countering Smell Cravings

One way to conquer this sensitivity of senses is to avoid going near places where there is food available. Make sure you aren't hungry when you leave home. Smelling food on a hungry stomach will test even the firmest resolve. Keep the windows up when you are driving past areas where there are fast food places or bakeries. As a last-ditch effort, chew some gum to change the flavor impulse from your mouth to mint (which is a food neutral taste) and turn up the volume on your car stereo.

When one sense is being overloaded, the other senses fade to prevent a stimuli breakdown. This is why people tend to turn the radio down when they are lost and are looking for a turn off they were supposed to take. It's because you can't concentrate when you are being overwhelmed in one sense area. Some cars even come with a standard feature to mute your car stereo when you shift the car into reverse. You can use this strategy to help you ignore smells when out and about. Likewise, you can do the same with your earphones when you have to walk past a food place where temptation lives.

Taste

Your sense of taste is equally important in controlling your cravings. If you smell something, the scent particles can move through the airways, touching the sensitive taste buds, which are nerve receptors on the tongue where we experience the five tastes of salty, sweet, sour, umami, and bitter. These nerve receptors are closely linked to the receptors that inform the thalamus where our emotions are formed in the brain.

So, when you eat something, you have an emotional experience to the taste of that food. Eating something sweet like chocolate may make you feel loved or give you a sense of belonging. Controlling your tastes and how these trigger appetite and cravings are also about controlling your emotions and being mindful of your emotional needs.

Sweet tastes are associated with positive emotions such as love, joy, belonging, and safety, while sour or salty tastes can be associated with negative emotions such as anger, jealousy, and hate. Your cravings can then tell you a bit about your emotional state. If you crave sweets, you need to feel loved. When you crave salty foods such as cheese and crackers or fried steak, you are feeling angry or upset about something.

Strategies for Countering Taste Cravings

Become aware of your emotional state with awareness activities such as writing, meditation, and developing your ability to self-gauge your feelings. Once you know how you feel, you will begin to understand a specific craving you may be having. Deal with the feeling before you try stuffing it with food.

If you are feeling angry, go for a walk or go hit a few rounds at the driving range until you feel your stress levels normalize. Don't just buy salty snacks because you are feeling upset and angry. They won't normalize your emotions. Beef jerky won't make you feel better.

Chewing gum helps to alleviate the cravings on your tongue, and you can try different flavor gums to help you manage cravings. If you have a craving for something, stay out of the supermarket or food district altogether. Instead, drink some water. A fuller stomach signals the brain that you are no longer in need of food, which lowers cravings.

When you plan your snacks, be sure to plan them according to your taste buds too. Just because you are following a healthier leaner diet doesn't mean your food needs to be boring. Explore exciting flavors with spices, herbs, and seeds that pop in your mouth. There is a big difference between the rice cakes I eat for lunch and some that I have seen my colleagues choking on. Mine aren't dry. They are loaded with goodness with lean slivers of meat, fresh and crispy lettuce, sesame seeds, poppy seeds (which are sweet), baby tomatoes, and crispy cucumber. One bite is pure heaven. I use my taste cravings to help me. I don't deny them or let them run all over the show like unruly children.

Sound

There is something exciting about the sound of a packet of chips opening, isn't there? Even animals respond to certain sounds with slavering tongues. I recently got my first dog

since childhood, and Max is a serious snacker (just like I was).
I can't open a packet in my house without him sitting right
next to me with expectation in his eyes. It's a great way to
make myself feel guilty so I won't snack uncontrollably.

There are certain sounds that we are programmed to feel
hungry upon hearing. Take the sound of meat hitting a hot
pan. Yip, that sizzling sound is quite intoxicating. What about
the sound of a soda being opened, food being sliced, popcorn
snapping in the pot, the plop of a lump of sugar in tea, the
crunchy grinding sound of that first bite into a large
hamburger, or the sound of blocks of chocolate being broken
off a bar? You've probably got your own sounds that trigger
your cravings and drive you quite mad. So, how do you
counter these auditory inspired cravings?

Strategies for Countering Sound Cravings

When you plan your meals, snacks, or indulge in a spoil, be
sure to do so with food that satisfies your sound cravings too.
Pay attention to the sound your food makes. Do you hear the
sizzle as you fry up some lean beef steaks in the skittle for
lunch over the weekend? Savor it. Perhaps you can focus on
the sound of a knife slicing through some whole grain bread
loaded with salads and turkey breast flakes? Zoom in your
ears, listening carefully to the sounds, letting them become
new triggers for sound cravings.

It is possible to replace certain harmful sound cravings with
more healthy sound effects of food, thereby reducing your
cravings. Sitting in a communal eating hall such as at a

cafeteria at work can be a real challenge when you hear your colleagues munching away at their huge burgers or cracking through some greasy fries. Strike up a conversation, or listen to some music on your earphones instead. Become aware of the sounds your own chewing makes. Savor each crunch.

Overall Strategies

Being strategy-wise is important to help you limit or banish your food cravings. You are fighting a war against your own nature, and you need to be prepared in all ways possible to keep temptation at bay. Here are some other great strategies on how to limit the ways in which your senses can lead you astray:

- **Don't Go Shopping With an Empty Stomach**

When you are hungry, the sight of food and any alluring smells and tastes will have a much greater hold on you. Science has proven that if you shop while hungry, you will be more likely to buy calorie-rich foods. Cornell's University conducted a study that proved participants who ate nothing before shopping were more likely to load up with calorie-rich foods in their baskets, while participants who had been told to eat crackers until they were full before going shopping were more likely to load up on low-calorie foods. If you are hungry, your body goes into starvation mode, and it hoards calories (Miller, 2019).

- **Try New Food Preparation Methods**

If your style of cooking is cumbersome and takes long, you will be doubly tempted to eat takeout or eat out. It's time to try new and different cooking methods and spice up your food preparation methods. When you cook with passion, you will be more inclined to want to eat at home, which already provides a lower calorie meal (if you cook wisely). Invite a few friends over who are also aware of your food decisions and will support you in your journey. Having support and encouragement will help you want to try new foods and new ways to cook. If you always fry your food, try to boil or bake it instead. Try new ingredients and different recipes that fall in line with your food plans.

- **Manage Your Blood Sugar Levels**

Your blood sugar levels are what triggers the hunger hormone, and they lead to that feeling of you could eat a whole farm (never mind a horse). When your blood sugar levels are low, you will struggle to say no to food temptations. This means you are exceptionally vulnerable to giving in to food cravings, and it can quickly lead to overeating. It is also why diets don't work. When your diet encourages starvation, it means your blood sugar will dip, causing cravings and intense hunger. This activates your primitive control mechanisms that tell your body to hoard food since there is a shortage. And voila—overeating happens!

Signs of low blood sugar levels include:

☐ Sweating
☐ Exhaustion

- ☐ Feeling shaky
- ☐ Tingly lips
- ☐ Irritability and anxiety

The catch with blood sugar levels is that they don't reset instantly. It's not like you can eat an apple and instantly feel less hungry. You have to wait for the chemicals and hormones in your body to equalize before you can feel full or sated. The fastest way to restore your blood sugar levels is with a glucose tablet. It only contains three to four grams of carbs, which is relatively low in calories. The idea is to boost your blood sugar, not to overload your system by eating a whole pizza with a side serving of a gallon of ice cream. By the time your hunger has subsided from eating, you have already bypassed your actual food requirement and you're probably stuffed like a Thanksgiving turkey.

- **Give Yourself Rules to Follow**

If you have to think about your diet plan to figure out what works for you, it is a losing battle you are fighting. Your food dependency has already decided by the time you make up your mind about the number of calories you could still eat today. Make things really simple with some rules that become your habits. Here are a few of mine:

I will not eat chocolate during the week.

I will not have a spoil meal three days in a row.

I will have a glass of water before every meal.

When I sit down to eat, I will decide how much I am going to eat BEFORE I start to eat.

It is okay to ask for a doggy bag at a restaurant, and I WILL give that food to someone who needs it more than me.

I will stop and breathe between each spoon or fork full of food.

- **Plan to Avoid Sensory Temptations**

When you have a problem with food and can't control how much you eat, it means you need to control your exposure to food and eating. This might mean never going to lunch or dinner with colleagues, never having alcoholic beverages when you do go out as this lowers your self-control and leaves you open to being influenced, or never looking at adverts or the menu in the restaurant. If you do have to go out, decide beforehand what you will be eating and stick to it.

Even when grocery shopping, be sure to have a list of what you need (not what you want) and stick to it religiously. Don't pack your trolley with your eyes or nose. Use your mind to decide what foods work for you and which you should avoid.

Fighting Food Cravings

The worst food opponent you'll face is your cravings. It is a strong-willed foe, and it will take all of your courage and knowledge to outwit and outlast your hunger pangs and that water-in-the-mouth sensation you get by even thinking of something tasty. There are a few ways to keep cravings under control:

- **Drink Enough Water**

When you are hydrated, it helps to maintain an even blood sugar level, which helps balance your hunger pangs. Thirst often masquerades as hunger, so drink some water before you think of eating.

- **Eat Dense Foods**

When food takes a bit longer to digest, it keeps you fuller for longer, minimizing your cravings. Getting enough protein in your diet is a surefire way to keep hunger away. Increasing your protein intake by 25% can reduce cravings by a whopping 60% (Bjarnadottir, 2016).

- **Put Your Mind Elsewhere**

By thinking of something else that is more pleasant when you are feeling hungry, you are diverting your attention away from the alleged hunger you feel now. This is why when you are really busy and have no time to think, you may go all day without eating and not even realize it or suffer from even a single hunger pang. When you sit all day and have nothing to do, you will soon be convinced you're starving to death.

When you are thinking of something else to keep your mind busy, your body will sort itself. Combine this with drinking a glass of water and you've got a powerful combination.

- **Eat What You Plan**

Often, you may plan to eat something and end up eating something else, which is probably higher in calories than your original plan. So, plan your meals and stick to that plan. Don't let your mind tell you that you're not in the mood for that particular meal. Your logic determines the terms and conditions here, not your emotional and hungry brain.

- **Combat Stress and Practice Mindfulness**

When we are stressed, our bodies tend to see this as a sign of danger, which means "eat up." The best thing to do is to handle your stress, not your plate. Take control of the things that stress you out and wear you down by being mindful of who you are and where you are.

- **Sleep on It**

When you are tired, your ability to resist cravings is lowered. Sleep is necessary for your body's different mechanisms and to gain mental awareness. You may end up eating without even thinking of what you are eating when you are tired. A lack of sleep can also cause a chemical imbalance, which can negatively impact hormone production in the body, causing false hunger.

The Replacement Fillers

With the power to choose comes the responsibility to do so. You know which foods are bad for you, and it's up to you to swap them with healthier alternatives. These healthy replacements fill you up and stop cravings in their tracks.

Consider the following replacement fillers and the poor food choices you can avoid:

- **Milk**

If you drink milk or use it in your cooking, try to opt for low-fat or skimmed or even fat-free milk if possible. Full cream milk is high in fats and, thus, calories.

- **Sugar**

Swap sugar-coated cereals for whole grain varieties for breakfast, opt for a sugar replacement (such as Stevia) instead of adding sugar to your tea or coffee, and sweeten your granola with some fresh fruits rather than sprinkling sugar over.

- **Breads**

Change bagels, white bread, and muffins for whole grain options. Avoid eating bread late at night, rather opting for a rice cake.

- **Sauces**

Be sure to swap creamy sauces for vegetable base sauces to cut back more calories and fats. If you make your own sauce at home, try to use olive oil and avoid other kinds of cooking oil. Your heart will thank you.

- **Cooking Methods**

Try to use your griddle pan more instead of the frying pan or prepare your meat over a coal fire (barbeque style) if you can, instead of having to use oils to fry meat. Veggies can be prepared like this too by wrapping them in cute little aluminum foil pouches instead of frying them in the pan.

- **Stop the Fizz**

Many people are addicted to fizzy sodas and these are always loaded with corn syrup, making them a massive calorie carrier. Swapping sodas for 100% pure fruit juice or spring water is a much better option.

- **Go for Healthy Snacks**

We all want to snack at some point, and if we go for a healthy snack option, we certainly can. Consider these snacks that are all under 100 calories each:

- ☐ Whole grain cheese and tomato toastie
- ☐ Apple, grapes, and pineapple fruit salad
- ☐ Smoked salmon and reduced soft cheese
- ☐ Baked beans on whole wheat toast

☐ Homemade popcorn without butter

You are not being eaten by your food. The choices of which stimuli you are listening to, seeing, or tasting are all yours. You can choose to look at a tempting snack or choose to look away. You can also intentionally distract your focus so you can choose foods that don't disappoint you. The human body can cause our cravings to spike, but it is in our power to take physical control of your decisions and their consequences with your food choices.

Chapter 6: How to Combat Psychological Influences

Food issues start in your mind. It is how you think about food, your relationship with food, and what food does for you. Being fat is often not a food issue. It's a mental issue, a delicate challenge between habits, hormones, and emotions. When you learn to understand your mind and its ability to change your life, you will begin to write the story of your life, and you can take it in any direction (or size) you want.

What You Think About Food

Your brain is one of the first things to develop during fetal gestation. It will also be the last thing to perish when you die. It is powerful and potent, and it can also ruin or save your life. You can direct your thinking, but you need to know how to do that.

Simply telling your brain you are fat and need to lose weight will not help you achieve your goals. Instead, your brain might only focus on the words "fat" and "lose," which could end up being understood as fat loser, causing you to feel negative about yourself. Your hormones can become unbalanced, causing you to eat more, and there begins the downward and ever-widening spiral of comfort eating and weight gain.

Control your thinking, direct it towards positive things, and your emotions will follow. Tension will lessen, and soon, your hormones will also come into alignment. In extreme cases, you may need medical intervention to help you balance your hormones. But don't be too quick to look for the solution in a pill. Instead, be the change you desire to see (to roughly paraphrase Gandhi).

Your brain, like the rest of your body, is a physical expression you can train. Here's some great ways to do that:

- **Practice Gratitude**

When you make gratitude part of your day, it brings awareness of the things you can be thankful for into your mind. This makes you more positive and productive. I think of this as "I can and I am."

- **Look on the Bright Side**

Try to maintain a focus on the positive things in life. Look for that silver lining in all things so you don't get mentally weighed down.

- **Accept Duality**

Things will not always be 100% the way you want them. When you start dieting, you will slip up and have boo-boo days. It is inevitable. Life is duality. You do well with your goals today, and tomorrow you trip up. Accept this, move on, do better. No gain comes from lamenting your weaknesses.

- **Use Affirmations When in Doubt**

Affirmations are powerful phrases that can help direct your thinking. It keeps you on track with your goals. Some examples include:

I am more than a chocolate bar.

My day is going well due to my positive spirit.

Every day I am taking control of my life.

- **Monitor Your Self-Talk**

What you think to yourself has power. If you are thinking you are weak-willed, chances are that your thinking will come true. Instead, think every day how amazing the progress is that you have made in your weight management plan.

- **Write Your Goals**

Setting goals is really important. Write them out. Plan how you will reach them and what you will achieve when you reach the line of your goals.

- **List Your Assets**

We tend to focus on loss or deficiency, and as a result, we often forget all the amazing things we've got going for us. List your assets. Create a list of all the things you do well and let this motivate you. You can list every single thing you do well and that is in your favor. Mine began with: I am happy. I am driven. I succeed at getting out of bed each morning. I made it to work today without thinking of food. (And the list continues on and on.)

State of Mind, Mind Your Plate

Eating healthier does amazing things for your mind. It makes you happy. There is something about eating a lovely salad with fresh tuna flakes and grated low-fat cheese that is simply satisfying. When you do eat healthy, you feel better, which makes you feel even better, so you eat more healthy. The result is an ever-improving upward spiral to health.

When you feel amazing, you have an improved mood, which stimulates your appetite towards healthier foods. Simply put, when you feel good, you eat good and you'd happily eat a lean turkey whole wheat sandwich instead of craving the dark roast with a side of buttery mash potatoes that depression might drive you towards.

It is, therefore, important to improve your mood as much as possible. Here are a few mood improving tips to help you get started:

- **Get up Earlier**

By getting up a little earlier each day, you can give yourself enough time to get your morning started peacefully instead of having to rush madly to get to where you need to go. This also gives you the time to prepare for your day, make healthy lunch packs or snack packs to get you through the day and deal with cravings. Getting up early is the gift of time.

- **Smile and Make Others Smile**

A smile has power. It really makes someone else light up. Just smile at the people in the cars around you as you are "stuck" in a traffic jam. Notice what a difference it makes. It gladdens the heart, which (corny as it sounds) helps you feel better and eat better.

- **Clean up Around Yourself**

I remember watching a show on TV years ago that featured reclusive people who lived in terrible hoarding homes. These people were the abject image of misery, and invariably, they were always massively obese as well. This taught me the value of cleaning up. When I eat a meal, I wash the plate afterwards, even if I could have done it later when I get home from work. I pack away things around my home, never leaving a mess around me. When you have a mess around yourself, you will become a mess inside yourself. Crowded and messy homes breed unhappy souls.

- **Write and Rejoice**

Record your victories. Take the time to write about each of your goals you've reached. Whether it's dropping a pound this week or managing to only stop for essential groceries and not emotional groceries, record them, and be sure to celebrate in a non-food way.

- **Walk**

Moving is great for your body and your mind. The goal shouldn't just be to lose weight but also to shed some mental pounds. When your body exercises (even slightly), your brain produces serotonin and endorphins, which make you feel better. By feeling better, you will eat better, building a chain of "better" links.

- **Remember Good Memories**

Photos have never been my fondest things to look at. I always looked at the pictures and wondered why I was so fat in each. Instead, I have learned not to look at myself in the photos, but to reflect on the happy memories they represent. Now, I see trips to the beach, visits to parks, and events in the town I grew up in. I see the happiness I felt, and I realize it wasn't tied to my body or my weight; my happiness was always inside.

- **Listen to Music**

Music is scientifically proven to improve moods. When I feel terrible because my cravings got the better of me, or maybe I just had way more stress at work than I can deal with, I always start by putting on some music. I may stroll around my living room listening to Sinatra crooning through the speakers and, suddenly, life doesn't seem all that bad.

- **Set the Mood**

Most people don't take care of themselves the way they should. And while this is a book about weight management, I am not referring to weight here. Instead, I am talking about how to do things that make your mood better. Men tend to be really bad at this. But even some ladies struggle. Try to enhance your senses in soothing ways. Light a candle, play nice music, dim the lights, and take yourself on a date of self-appreciation. This might include massaging your own feet or, if you have some body massage gizmo, you could use that.

- **Spread "Nice"**

Doing nice things for other people spreads the cheer of giving. By actively trying to make other people's lives a little better, your own might improve dramatically.

- **Sleep**

Improve your mood by catching up on some Zs. Make sure to get at least seven to nine hours of sleep a night as this ensures you are well rested and able to handle life's challenges.

Stress and Hormones

Life is stressful. There's no way to argue that point, and the reality is that stress, if left unmanaged, can be a killer. It affects your heart health, and it also messes with your brain and the delicate balance of neurotransmitters and hormones that your body is regulated by.

When you are stressed, it triggers an increased production of the hormone cortisol, which is known as the stress hormone. Now, cortisol may have served a purpose in the prehistoric age where it boosted muscle tone and triggered the release of adrenaline, which made you run faster (requiring more energy) to avoid a serious threat (like a saber-toothed tiger), but today, there are no tigers. You don't have to run for your life, and the jungle is now concrete. Yet, this process still happens, and as a result, your brain believes you need to replace energy reserves you're about to burn while running away from that ancient predator. So, you are triggered to eat. The trigger was stress.

Needing energy and needing it quickly to evade the predator your brain thinks is hunting you, your brain will push you towards eating the highest sources of energy around you such as sweets. Not sure what this looks like? Just think of people who experience a sudden and traumatic experience. They start to shake, which is the effect of adrenaline burning through the energy stored in the muscles. When people suffer trauma or shake, the common cure is to take some glucose water to counter the sudden drop in blood sugar levels.

This is why when you are stressed or suffer trauma, you will have massive cravings for sweets or sugary treats. Overeating is also the brain's defense against what it perceives as high-energy lifestyles. Stress can lead to addictions in food consumption, drugs, and other habits.

Stress reduces the rate of calorie burn, causing a positive energy balance, which equates to weight gain. Therefore, stress slows down your metabolism, causing mass gain and lower energy consumption as your body tries to hoard resources for the perceived stressful situation (a threat according to your primitive brain) that you may be in (Yau and Potenza, 2013).

Beating Emotional Eating

Knowing that your biology is programmed to eat more when you are stressed or emotional is key in taking control. Your subconscious systems need to be taken off autopilot and you need to start actively making decisions and being in control.

The best way to head off emotional eating is to know your triggers and be aware when they appear so you can consciously make better decisions. Stress lowers blood sugar, which is what causes triggers to become internalized, and this is what causes you to eat when you really shouldn't need to. So, if you can regulate your blood sugar, you don't need to listen to those triggers as they have lost their survival value to your primitive brain. Thus, you no longer need to eat.

By reducing the symptoms of stress, you can also improve your blood sugar. So, when you are feeling stressed, take a walk (to release some endorphins), drink some water (to cool down), breathe mindfully (to slow the faster breathing brought on by stress), and think about other soothing things (to relax your mind).

Therefore, emotional eating is really your body's way to deal with the stress you are feeling, which it mistakenly interprets as your body being threatened, kicking the fight-or-flight system into overdrive. Emotional eating is more accurately called stress eating then.

Luckily, there's hope. Try these techniques to help you stop emotional or stress eating:

- **Mental Distraction**

When you are feeling stressed and the cravings start, it is a good idea to try some mental distraction first. You can do this by listing the colors of the cars around you, counting backwards from 50, naming the sounds you hear, giving names to the textures you feel around you, and finding descriptions for the scents you smell. This is an exercise in mindfulness.

- **Box Breathe**

Anxiety and stress often interrupts your body's normal breathing processes. You can easily reset these with a breathing exercise such as the box breathing method taught to law enforcement officers in the U.S. It's very simple.

Breathe in for a count of four, hold for a count of four, breathe out for a count of four, hold for a count of four, and repeat this four times. This is sure to slow your heart rate and cool your body while giving your mind something other than stress (or food) to think about by counting breaths.

- **Postcard Thoughts**

Negative thinking goes hand in hand with stress. However, instead of judging yourself or your thinking, imagine these thoughts like postcards you briefly view in the curio shop of your mind. Absently look at the thought, then let it go as if you are mailing it out to an unnamed destination in the world.

- **Journal**

When you write about your stressors, you reduce their power over you. It is an ideal way to express your feelings, come to terms with them, and take the power to choose your actions instead of being a victim who simply dives head first into a bowl of pastrami to hide from painful feelings.

- **Express Yourself With Art**

Art is a soothing way to deal with emotions, feelings, and thoughts. Draw, paint, and sculpt your way to inner peace and your stomach will thank you.

- **Ground Yourself**

We can all do with a reminder to relax. I have a set of ancient prayer beads I was given by a student that I now carry with me. The round beads are well-worn, and they remind me to take things easier. Having a tactile reminder such as a memory stone, a rosary, or some other meditative object is a great way to remind yourself of your physical existence and how your mind can and should be in sync with this.

- **Identify What Your Trigger Is**

Each of us have something that triggers our emotional eating binges. If you know your enemy, you can defeat it. So, if you are bored and this causes hunger, phone someone instead of slicing that apple pie. If you are angry, go pull up weeds in your garden, and if you are sad, go cry on a friend's shoulder.

Emotional eating can be beaten if you arm yourself with knowledge, skills, strategies, and have the will to take action to stop being a victim of your primitive biology, your blood sugar levels, and your own feelings.

This Is My Body, It Is Real

I've managed to lose weight and reach my goal weight. Note I say "goal weight" and not "ideal weight." This is because we have very twisted ideas about how much we should weigh and what we should look like. In most people's books, I am still too fat. In my book, I am at a size that is comfortable, healthy, and most importantly, I am happy.

We are given this twisted view on what we "should" weigh by social media. Our body image is all wrong due to a proliferation of pictures of skinny ladies and buff and brawny guys who are all "living the dream." The reality is that those photos are often digitally altered, they show people who have possibly had all manner of body altering surgeries, and they don't show the other 500 photos that were taken that showed fewer desirable views of the person in question.

Real people don't look like this.

Trying to emulate a false image of perfection is the start to eating disorder hell. Girls end up being anorexic, and guys end up bulking to gym but get flabby results instead. Find what is the real and "ideal" for your body and for your lifestyle. Be real, be you!

Chapter 7: How to Combat Social Influences

Everywhere we look, we see food. It is such an integral part of Western society that I struggle to imagine a world where we don't see food adverts every five seconds. Is the world really that hungry? Or, are we simply being conditioned to fit into a highly integrated money-making machine? We eat (spending money), get fat, go on diets (spending more money), lose weight (supporting social media when we brag about our success), only to see more food ads, and gain weight to continue the cycle.

In our modern world, we can't ignore or underestimate the role of social influences on our weight management journey. Doing so sets us up for failure. Be conscious of how you use social media, the influence it has on you and on your family, and how it can begin to brainwash you in a subtle manner if you let it.

How Society Fills Us Up

When we are being inundated from every angle by words, images, phrases, and a popularization of food, it is hard to stay on the right track with your food choices. When you have a family to care for it can be even harder to stay the course towards a healthy and nutritious lifestyle. Your family influences you with their choices and wants with food, but you can also influence them. This can take some careful planning and strategies like the following:

- **Control What Food Enters Your Home**

When your home is a junk food-free zone, it is much easier to stay on track. However, if you buy junk food and hide it in the cupboard, you aren't hiding it from your mind, which will tell you at three in the morning how hungry you are and that you need a snack on the half a jar of Nutella you hid away.

Don't allow foods that are bad for you into your home. This is your first line of defense. No matter what advertisements you see, don't indulge things out of curiosity when you know they are bad for you.

- **Encourage Choice**

If you have a family to care for, you want to avoid seeming like a food dictator. You can't be the hummus Hitler of your family. Allow your family to choose what they eat and how much they eat, knowing that you have controlled the food that is in your house. So, your family can select from the foods you have chosen, but don't let them force or coerce you into buying things you know are bad just because they want to choose it.

With choices, you should involve your family in the meal decisions. Give your family healthy options to choose from: "Would you like some brown rice with steamed salmon and crisp veggies followed by dessert of apple slices with nut butter and a dark chocolate drizzle?" Sell the food choices to your family. Don't use words like "low-fat" or "low-calorie" when speaking about their meals as your family will not appreciate these words. Simply put, they don't sound appetizing.

Healthy food can be sexy if you use the right words, an appealing presentation, and give your family the right to choose what they would like to eat (from YOUR pantry).

- **Form Healthy Eating Traditions**

When you simply gobble your meals in front of the TV, you are not eating healthy (no matter what is on your plate). Encourage your family to eat at the dining room table. Give each family member a task to include them in the meal ritual. Your younger children can set the table and the older children can carry the food to the table while you can help to dish up while your children can tell you the size of their portions. Not all children will want to eat everything you make, so give them a limited choice. Perhaps you can even make a game out of it. Allow your children one food they don't have to eat, so they get to choose between a couple of foods that they aren't necessarily too happy with. Be sure to still make a food group they do enjoy eating too.

Encourage your family to talk about good topics at the dinner table and set the example by talking about fun things, not politics or religion or money, at the table. Be sure to keep an eye that your family stops to breathe and listen and eat in small bites while the meal is ongoing. Meals shouldn't be rushed.

- **Share Goals**

If you want to lose some weight, then you can share your goals with your family. If you have been eating willy-nilly, then chances are that your family have also been suffering with weight issues. If you share your goals, then your children and partner will lose weight in proportion to your own weight loss battles.

- **Control the View**

If you constantly see things that aren't healthy to eat, you will find your resolve to eat healthy crumble. Appeal to your and your family's food interests by placing healthy snacks in easy viewing range. This means you could add colored apples, fresh berries, bright orange oranges, and crispy sprigs of celery to the displays in your kitchen. Feast your eyes healthily and your body will follow.

- **Sync Your Salt**

By removing the salt shaker from the table, you lower the need for unnecessary salts. People have a tendency to add salt to their food without even tasting whether their food needs it. Encourage your family to enjoy the natural taste of food, not the pop of salty food. You can also try alternative food types such as beetroot salt (which is an organic mineral salt), Himalayan pink salt, and other kinds of salt.

- **Dish up at the Pot**

This may seem rude, but don't take all the food you have prepared to the table. This encourages people to eat past the point of being sated. Rather ladle up smaller portions, talk for a while at the table, and if someone is really still hungry, they can then have another half a serving of some food. Don't encourage eating after the taste. Be sure not to overcook either.

- **Keep Meals Regular**

By having regular meal times with your family (and even with yourself alone), you can develop a healthy routine. Eventually, you will choose a healthy alternative without much thought required. It will become your habit.

Following a schedule will also help you plan when snacks are acceptable. You may have a rule of not eating snacks 90 minutes before a main meal to keep appetites up. With young or active children, you may need to be a little more flexible, but you can fix this challenge by having healthy small snacks available for them to enjoy. Having little packets of homemade trail mix (dried fruits and nuts) is a great way to allow a healthy snack.

- **Listen to Your Family**

If your child tells you they are full and don't want to eat more, then listen. Don't be a feeder who insists on their children eating all of their food (when the plate is overfull). Instead, let your children tell you they are no longer hungry. You can also keep their plate until later, giving them the option to eat the food they weren't interested in earlier. Your child won't starve from pecking at one or two meals, so don't force-feed them.

You can inform and teach your family, and you don't have to lose the war against overeating just because you've been doing things the wrong way till now. Be the change you desire in your family. Educate them, making them aware of food and their lives. Remember that they won't want a food dictator, so give your family choices, but firmly choose to limit the role of unhealthy food in your home.

Becoming a Social Influencer

We humans are social creatures. It is no secret that we love to hang out together, eat meals together, and be generally social around our food. If someone invites you over to their house, it is tradition to ask what you can bring. This is a sharing tradition that probably goes back all the way to the early caveman who would almost certainly bring food to a prospective mate.

Become a social influencer by arranging fun social events that aren't focused on food. Come up with games nights, get friends to go bowling with you (preferably somewhere that there isn't a restaurant or bar), or make Saturdays about hiking and enjoying a healthy picnic after. Here are some other amazing ideas of being social without eating or drinking alcohol:

- **Go Biking or Hiking**

Getting physically active together is a great way to hang out. While this can work up quite an appetite, you can play into this by catering healthy treats to eat afterwards. Picnic lunches tend to be more health conscious too, which helps.

- **Do Something Creative Together**

When you and your friends or family do something creative together, you gain entertainment and excitement from something other than food. You can combine this with making healthy snacks and perhaps making your own treats using colorful veggies, fruits, nuts, and seeds.

- **Travel**

Instead of going to a restaurant, pack a healthy basket with appropriate snacks and take your friends or family on a drive down the coast or up a mountain. Travel and spend time together instead of gaining weight together.

- **Attend a Concert**

Going to a live concert can be one of the best forms of entertainment to enjoy together with your friends, and it doesn't involve food, nor does it have to involve alcohol.

- **Get Grounded**

Take up gardening! Get your family to support you in making a beautiful feature garden, laying out a path, or planting seedlings. If you live in a small apartment, you can always do a mini-garden using an assortment of pots. Veggie gardens are an excellent way to get into growing your own food too.

- **Renovate Something**

Instead of spending a fortune on hiring a contractor, involve your family and some friends and do some renovating at home. This can be a great way to have fun together and get a sense of accomplishment.

Social Hunger Scales

Educate your friends or family on hunger, food, and cravings. This may not seem like the most socially acceptable topics, but these are essential for helping others understand the choices you are making. You might also be surprised by how many people will support you and be curious to learn more.

Social events, like going to a restaurant, are often challenging to someone on a restrictive or health conscious diet. A good way to keep yourself on track is to use a hunger scale. If you are 60% hungry, you can decide to only eat 60% of your plate. This can extend to deciding BEFOREHAND whether you want a dessert or not. Social pressure is to always eat with your friends, to have what they are having.

By discussing your hunger scale with friends, you can help them make better decisions about how much to order at a restaurant, and it opens up other more interesting options for dining out. I have a group of close friends who all understand and support my hunger scale method. We have gotten into the habit of deciding on which dishes look good at restaurants, and then we order only half the food we'd eat, mixing and sharing. This allows us to sample a larger portion of food from the menu without actually each eating a whole plate.

If I do have to go to a restaurant where I know the portions will be big, I ask for a doggy bag beforehand so I can scoop out extra food before I start eating. This removes the temptation to eat more than I can and should.

The hunger scale is something that was created by the Derbyshire Community Health Services. There are 10 levels on the hunger scale with number one being so hungry that you are dizzy and feel faint and have to lie down since you are weakened by low blood sugar levels. On the other end of the scale, at number 10, you feel stuffed as if you just had Christmas lunch and two helpings of dessert. Here's how it works:

Level one to three: Extremely hungry and your body is weakened, needing food. When you feel like your hunger is at this scale, you should eat enough food to be filled. This will probably be a whole plate of food.

Level four to six: You feel hungry, you think about food, or you are slightly hungry and could eat a little. On this level of the scale, you can eat a modest or small meal, topping up your calorie consumption just enough to be sated.

Level seven to ten: You feel full, but your eyes tell you to eat a little more, although you don't need it. You might also feel completely stuffed, not wanting to even think about food. At this level of the scale, you shouldn't eat at all.

To use the hunger scale, you sit quietly before your meal, thinking about your body, sensing the feeling in your stomach. Has it been three to five hours since your last meal? There should be a slight cramping or empty feeling in your stomach area, indicating your stomach is empty and needs food. If you feel the hunger in your mouth or any other part of your body, you are emotional eating.

While eating, also listen to the things your body is telling you. Eat slowly, allowing the signals of your brain to catch up to the chemicals in your digestive tract. When you start to feel full, stop eating. Don't feel obliged to "clean your plate" or "not waste food." You are full, and that is enough.

The reality is you will only enjoy the food while you are between a three and a six on the scale. Below three, you are eating for survival; above seven you are stuffing food into an already full tank.

Cultivating Better Time Management for Eating

"I'm fine with making my diet commitments at home during the weekends, but when I'm at work I forget to eat or I don't have time to. Then I am ravenous when I'm driving home, and the temptation to grab some burgers and fries is just too big!" A friend of mine recently complained bitterly that she just couldn't keep her blood sugar levels stable. As a result, she was healthy over weekends, but in the week, she failed miserably. There just didn't seem to be time for healthy eating when she was at work.

Time management is not just about making sure you get up early in the morning and pack a healthy lunch, it is also about managing your time carefully while at work so you get to eat that lunch (and not gobble it down). This is a skill that is sadly lost during the busy work week.

124

To keep your health goals, eat your lunch, and balance your mental and hunger levels, you need to make time to eat calmly. Lunch can't be a situation of quickly grabbing that lovely whole wheat sandwich you made and stuffing it down in three bites while you continue typing a report for the CEO. That's not lunch, that's a force feed.

Look at the activities of the day. Note which activities are most important. These need to be done first thing in the morning as you are freshest mentally and your blood sugar levels are more stable if you eat a healthy breakfast. Towards 11 o'clock, you might begin to feel a level four to five on the hunger scale, and you may want to eat. If you can have a break, great. Have your lunch. If you can't, this is where a healthy snack comes in.

Usually, this is the time I snap open a trail mix packet, shaking some goodness into my mouth, and as a bonus, the crunch wakes me up a little too. This lifts my hunger level back up to a six or seven on the hunger scale. I can last a few more hours if I have to. Ideally, I will eat my lunch around one pm.

I take my lunchtime. It is as important to me as any other task of the day. Whether I only take 30 minutes to walk to the local park or I go sit by the fountain in the plaza, I leave my desk (and my work) and I go enjoy my meal. I eat slowly, breathing between each bite. I chew carefully, allowing my mouth to do its job of masticating my food, ensuring the right mix of enzymes are present in my food as it reaches my stomach.

In the past, I used to find I packed too much lunch, and would struggle to eat the last few bites, but now I know better, and I pack just enough to satisfy my hunger, but not so much that I end up on a level 10 of the hunger scale. Nobody can work on that Christmas-feel stomach, so don't.

Returning to my office, I am able to work more efficiently, my blood sugar levels are more equalized, and they remain consistent thanks to the low GI foods I focus on for lunch. I manage to do the remaining tasks for my day before I leave work for the day. If I have a few minutes, I may sit and prepare my diary for the next day, making sure I know what lies ahead. If it is a very stressful day, I will make sure to pack more smaller snack packs. This means that even if I have to skip lunch, I can still keep my blood sugar levels balanced and stop cravings.

Teaching Family About Misinformation

"Why don't you just take this new pill I heard about?" My brother was being helpful, as usual. However, I had heard this before. "It's amazing! You take one in the morning and you won't have cravings, and best of all, you can eat all you like, but you will still lose weight." Sounds too good to be true? It is.

I have had to educate many a well-meaning friend or family member about the absolute flood of misinformation and health fraud that circulates on social media and in the press. It can be quite the minefield to find a supplement or dietary substitute that works. So, I don't. I go for what is real, organic, and medically proven to work.

There are so many food fads, health gimmicks, diet tricks, and other crazy ideas about healthy eating out there that have no basis in fact that I have to be careful, and I encourage my friends and family to also be careful. The human body is not something to trifle with.

Here's a quick guide to keep you on the right path and spot misinformation:

- **It's Too Good to Be True**

When you read something and it sounds miraculous, it's probably a fad or a fake. At best, it costs you a bit of money. At worst, it costs you your health when your kidneys suddenly fail.

- **Quick Results "You Can Believe"**

When it comes to weight loss, it's not about how fast you get it off. It's about how you are able to keep it off. Rush diets will not help you change your overeating lifestyle. You can't sustain those kinds of efforts, and they are not healthy. Slow and steady progress is what you want.

- **Too Simple**

Dieting isn't simple. It's complicated, and it requires that you know about things like calories, energy balance, calorie intake versus thermodynamic burn of these in the body, and a host of other strange terms. Even if you don't want to delve into that much detail, you should be aware that the scientists and dieticians who design a diet have done the thinking for you, and that their results are medically proven with long-term case studies, peer reviews, and numbers that prove their conclusions. I have even seen one diet that promised results based on a trial involving nine patients! Nine patients! How could that possibly be a trial? Check information, question findings, and make up your own mind.

- **Simplified Lists of Food**

Food is not your enemy. I'm not going to say you should never eat potatoes again in your life. Instead, I know from experience that it takes balance, moderation, and body awareness to reach your goal weight and stay there. Along the way, you can indeed eat some of the foods you like, but always in moderation and with awareness of the hunger scale. So, be wary of articles that cite food as being "good" or "bad."

- **"Highly Satisfied Customers"**

Oh, I hate seeing this on a product or diet write up. Everything under the sun has highly satisfied customers. Even bin bags have highly satisfied customers. Everything also has highly unsatisfied customers. It doesn't do squat for research though. And when a product plays the celeb card, where they point to some low-time celeb who has used their dieting pill, powder, syrup, or contraption with "huge success," I am quick to shove it back onto the shelf.

Be real! Even if some celeb is using this particular product, they are also using a personal fitness trainer, starving themselves, or only eating cabbage all day to look as "good" as they do. It's social media eating your soul. Get real! That product won't solve your problems because your problem isn't just overeating. Your weight challenges are based on your biology, hormones, food culture, and mental framework. How will a pill fix all of that?

Ultimately, your health, your goal weight, and your thinking paradigm about your weight and your food habits is what you should be focusing on, not the latest fad, social media craze, or public opinion.

Chapter 8: How to Combat Habitual Eating

Many people eat what they do because it has become their habit. They choose subconsciously to eat foods that tip the scales in the favor of weight gain. This is not something people think about. Instead, it is a habit they have formed or even inherited from their primary caregivers that simply runs their lives. Pretty soon, that habit can ruin their lives.

Munching Habits

Whenever you start to eat something without thinking about it, you have activated a food habit. These habits are often tied to places, people, events, and emotions. So, if you always eat a chocolate bar when you watch a sad movie, that is a food habit. If you always eat pasta with extra cream in the sauce when Johnny visits, then that is a food habit. And if you always raid the fridge after speaking with your mom who keeps asking when you will finally have a boyfriend/girlfriend, then that is a food habit.

Note that none of these food habits have anything to do with being hungry or meeting the needs of your hunger. Instead, you eat for the sake of food, for the sake of habit, and for the emotional need you may temporarily be feeling.

There isn't even any thought that goes into it. Like breathing, as soon as a trigger happens (the movie starts, Johnny shows up, or mom calls), you are ready to fulfill the habit. It is, in essence, mindless eating.

Identifying Bad Food Habits

If you want to change something, you need to acknowledge it first. You have to know your enemy, and it's you! Your habits are responsible for your weight gain. Only when you know when, where, why, and how you pursue bad eating habits can you begin to change for the better.

Identifying your bad food habits starts with awareness. Remember, you are engaging in these habits almost subconsciously. You need to bring your habits into the light so you can see, know, and defeat them.

Start by keeping a food diary. Write down everything you eat from the moment you wake up to the moment you go to sleep. Record portion size, what is on the plate, how you felt before the meal, what you felt after the food was consumed, and how you rated on the hunger scale before the meal.

You may be quite surprised by meals and snacks you didn't know you were having. After all, your body is quite capable of taking over and opening a fridge or loading up a plate. Before you know it, you are slipping into culinary coercion.

Try these following tips to help you notice typically bad eating habits and begin to take ownership of them so you can make changes for the better:

- **Eating in Front of the TV**

A really unhealthy habit people have is to sit in front of the TV after dinner and snack while channel hopping. You are distracted by the TV, and before you know it, you've delved through a half a pound bag of chips or candy.

Rather keep some healthy snacking options handy if you know you get the munchies when you're watching TV. Consider having some crisp celery sticks with Greek yogurt and digestive biscuits handy. Make sure to only take out as much as you need to eat based on your hunger scale. Don't sit there with the whole box or packet ... you know you will eat them all!

If you still crave eating in front of the TV, then rather switch off the TV and call someone you care about, have a Zoom call, or fill in a crossword puzzle. Keep active so your mind won't turn to food.

- **Irregular Eating Times**

Your body goes into crisis mode when it doesn't know when your next meal will be. It instantly believes the drought has struck, and it needs to hoard resources to survive. By keeping regular hours, and eating consistently at the same time, you increase your body's comfort and destress. As a result, you will eat less, and you will be more aware of your place on the hunger scale.

Try to eat regular meals instead of snacking non-stop. This will help your blood sugar remain steady, which will aid in reducing cravings. Have healthy snack alternatives handy in case you do feel yourself dip into the six to one number on the hunger scale.

Keep busy so you don't turn to snacks out of boredom.

- **Relying Too Much on Takeout**

It is certainly more convenient to stop for a ready-to-eat takeout meal than heading home after a long day and having to spend an hour in the kitchen making dinner for your family. However, if this becomes your habit more than it is the exception to the rule, you have developed a really bad food habit.

Break the habit of fast food buying and do a little preparation instead. If you know you will have a long day at work, then precook something for dinner that morning or the night before. You can also pre-cut some veggies, place meat in the slow cooker to simmer on its own, and you can make extra meals that you freeze and only need to heat for when you need them. These are all healthier than takeout.

Make cooking a communal activity so you not only think of cooking as producing food but also see it as producing memories. Your children can participate in preparing foods, and you will find it a pleasant use of time.

- **Being Unable to Waste Food**

Cooking isn't an exact science, and when you have a family, it becomes more of a volatile experiment. What little Jimmy ate last week he will hate this week, and the same goes for your spouse who decides not to eat all of their food. If you were raised in a home that was poor, you may have an aversion to wasting food. The end result of this could be to eat more than you intend to. It isn't wrong to waste food if it means you don't gain weight. Rather cook more so you have enough to put food away for a second meal that you keep in the freezer.

Teach your children not to put more in their plates than they can eat, and remind them they can always ask for seconds if they really are still hungry.

- **Sweet Snacks All Week Long**

Some office spaces offer teatime treats on the house with muffins, cupcakes, biscuits, and cakes. Instead of eating these all week long, you can rather save them for one day a week such as having Friday pie day. In the scheme of things, this would reduce your sweets intake dramatically as opposed to eating sweets all week long.

Sweet cravings are often due to being lonely. So, when you feel cravings hit, don't jump to the habitual "stuff your face with candies" routine. Instead, invite some friends over for a chat, go out to walk in the park, or take up a hobby.

- **Our Daily Bread**

Bread is a staple food that many people rely on at least one meal a day. If you feel a little peckish, you automatically grab a slice of bread or a bagel instead of eating some fruits or nuts. This is a major habit that has wide ranging negative side effects. Break the bread habit by only having enough bread in the house for one day, or buy extra but freeze the slices or rolls for later use.

Replace breads with similar but healthier alternatives such as rice cakes or crackers so you don't instantly miss the comfort of starchy breads.

- **Sweet Agony**

Most people have an addiction to sugar. Quite simply put, we crave the high we get from the carbs in sugary sweets. The mere crinkling of papers is enough to turn heads and make mouths salivate. It is one of the worst food habits to cultivate, and if you can't go a day or a week without eating candy, you are in serious trouble.

You need to shift your thinking, and when you want to reach for candy, you should grab a fruit instead. Why not have a few sweet grapes instead of toffees? Can't you have some apple slices with peanut butter for a snack instead of eating a chocolate bar?

The real sweetness you crave might be company or friendship. So, don't put your energies into a bad habit when you could be out there making friends.

- **Hab-butter**

Many people can't eat food without spreading butter all over it. This is so extreme that they look offended if they eat at your home and there's no butter on the table. Yet, butter is extremely bad for your health, and it's high in fat, which is carb rich and leads to excess calories and weight gain. Worst of all, people don't even know how much butter they use because it's not like they measure it.

Replace butter with low-fat options like plant-based margarines or spread. Most breads don't need butter to moisten them. You can add tomatoes, cucumbers, and lettuce to make a juicy sandwich. When you do decide to change your habit, you may find your brain conveniently "forgets" not to put butter on your bread. You can either throw out all butter, or you need to label it with reminders to yourself that you are only allowed to butter toast in the morning, and the rest of the day you must eat your food without butter (for example).

Routine and Good Eating Habits

Now that you are aware of the bad eating habits you have and how you should change them, it's important to look at good eating habits you may need to cultivate. These habits are there to keep you on track and maintain your body while you deal with the real issues that drive you to food.

There is no quick fix. Instead, you are slowly rebuilding or growing yourself to be who you are capable of being—a healthy and happy person.

Consider these tips on healthy routines and good eating habits:

- **Start Small and Start Slow**

Rome wasn't built in one day, and you're not going to turn into a vegan who magically loses 150 pounds in a month overnight. Drastic changes may seem inspiring, but it's small changes that become new routines that carry us through to victory. If you want to leave off a bad habit such as eating extra bread, then do so by reducing the amount of bread you eat, followed by changing it to an alternative to bread that is more healthy. Don't try to leave out a bad habit completely from the start. Dramatic changes don't last. Wise, well-thought through and incremental changes do.

- **Practice Mindfulness**

One of the biggest problems with bad food habits is that we don't think. We are off on another planet (usually our emotional pity party planet) as we habitually stuff a second helping of bagels with extra butter into our mouths. Become present in your life. Notice how you feel, what you are doing, what you want to do, and why.

Mindfulness slows things down in a hectic world so you can actually think. Simply breathe in between bites as you eat your meal. Savor the tastes, and let your body enjoy the sustenance you are eating.

- **Go Small**

When it comes to serving food, go small. Stop using large bowls, plates, or cutlery. If you reduce the size of your plates, you will automatically serve smaller size servings, which will help you eat less, and you can then clean your plate without feeling guilty about eating too much food.

- **Prepare for Healthy Cravings**

While you want to say you don't snack and that you don't get midnight cravings, the reality is that you probably will get those "bad" cravings for a while as you settle into your new routines and good eating habits. So, prepare healthy options. Surround yourself with healthy snack foods, and make sure to throw unhealthy food out. Temptations that are hard to resist should be kept at a distance. Just like an alcoholic who can't have alcohol in their house, you should avoid having bad food in your house.

Time Savers for cooking and Preparation

When cooking and preparing meals, it is popular to make meals ahead of time, batch cook, pack meals in individual portions, and prepare ingredients beforehand. If you are unsure of what foods to put into a meal or how to structure the week's menu, you can download a suitable app like WW (Weight Watchers Reimagined).

Prepare on a regular time schedule. If you cook at four, then do so every day. If you are doing batch cooking, then stick to the rule of having one item in the oven and two items on the stove top at the same time as more only leads to chaos and disaster. Be organized in your prep to make sure you have all the required ingredients and make sure to plan which areas of the kitchen are for which recipes you are busy making. Save more time by having a grocery list pad that you hang from the fridge door (or an app that you update on your mobile). Not having an accurate grocery list leads to splurge buying and wastes your time.

Conclusion

If you are challenged by weight issues, it is not the food that's the problem. Food is the symptom. Bigger issues are the ways in which you think about food, how you have been conditioned to include food into your culture, lifestyle, and habits.

This book has equipped you with everything you need to successfully change your food lifestyle. In Chapter 1 to Chapter 4, you learned about the physiological, psychological, social, and habitual reasons you aren't able to control your eating. It was an eyeopener, wasn't it?

Chapter 5 to Chapter 8 helped you form some strategies that are realistic, easily implemented, and effective at putting you back in the pilot's seat while taking your life off autopilot. You are now in control, possibly for the first time in your life.

Here is my wish for you, dear reader:

I wish for you to always be present and mindful in your life, to enjoy your meals, to have a deep reverence for the life you sustain through eating, and to feel empowered to make wise and healthy decisions for your life and your body. It will not always be easy, but it is within your reach, and you can grasp the life you were meant to live.

Your weight loss journey starts here, and you finally have all the skills you need to walk this road successfully. I wish you

well and encourage you to educate others as you walk ahead
with a lighter and healthier body each day.

References

Andrews, R. (2021). *All about energy balance.* Precision Nutrition. https://www.precisionnutrition.com/all-about-energy-balance

Bayliss, J. (2014). *How family influence eating habits – and your friends too!* Jennie Bayliss. https://www.jenniebayliss.com/family-influence-eating-habits/

Bjarnadottir, A. (2016). *11 Ways to stop cravings for unhealthy foods and sugar.* Healthline. https://www.healthline.com/nutrition/11-ways-to-stop-food-cravings

Carter, E. Watts, P. (2016). *The science of hunger and what makes us 'hangry.'* Independent. https://www.independent.co.uk/life-style/health-and-families/features/science-hunger-and-what-makes-us-hangry-a6828111.html

Centers for Disease Control and Prevention. (n.d.). *Childhood obesity facts.* CDC. https://www.cdc.gov/obesity/data/childhood.html#:~:text=Prevalence%20of%20Childhood%20Obesity%20in%20the%20United%20States&text=For%20children%20and%20adolescents%20aged,to%2019-year-olds.

Geng, L. (2011). *You are (as smart as) what you eat.* Pursuit of Research. https://pursuitofresearch.org/2011/02/09/you-are-as-smart-as-what-you-eat/

Gray, N. (2011). *Poor childhood diet linked to low IQ, suggests study.* Food Navigator. https://www.foodnavigator.com/Article/2011/02/08/Poor-childhood-diet-linked-to-low-IQ-suggests-study

Gwinn, A. (2019). *Are your friends making you fat?* AARP. https://www.aarp.org/health/healthy-living/info-2019/friends-influence-eating-habits.html

Magill, A. (2018). *What is the relationship between food and mood?* Mental Health First Aid. https://www.mentalhealthfirstaid.org/external/2018/03/relationship-food-mood/

Martinali, J. (2019). *Consumers' food choices and emotions.* Behavioral Research Blog. https://www.noldus.com/blog/consumers-food-choices-and-emotions

Miller, E. (2019). *Why you shouldn't grocery shopping on an empty stomach.* Infogrocery. https://infogrocery.com/avoid-grocery-shopping-empty-stomach

Nursekey. (n.d.). *Cultural and religious influences on food and nutrition.* Nursekey.

https://nursekey.com/cultural-and-religious-influences-on-food-and-nutrition/

Luca, F., Perry, G. H., & Di Rienzo, A. (2010). Evolutionary adaptations to dietary changes. *Annual Review of Nutrition, 30,* 291–314. https://doi.org/10.1146/annurev-nutr-080508-141048

Robinson, L. & Smith, M. (n.d.). *Social media and mental health.* Help Guide. https://www.helpguide.org/articles/mental-health/social-media-and-mental-health.htm

Savage, J. S., Fisher, J. O., & Birch, L. L. (2007). Parental influence on eating behavior: conception to adolescence. *The Journal of law, medicine & ethics : a journal of the American Society of Law, Medicine & Ethics,* 35(1), 22–34. https://doi.org/10.1111/j.1748-720X.2007.00111.x

SportMedBC. (n.d.). *How a workplace can impact your eating habits.* SportMedBC. https://sportmedbc.com/article/how-workplace-can-impact-your-eating-habits

Truth About Weight. (n.d.). *How hormones steer our appetite and eating behaviour.* Truth About Weight. https://www.truthaboutweight.global/global/en/science/how-hormones-steer-our-appetite-and-eating-behaviour.html

University of California San Francisco. (2019). *Obesity*. USCF (benioffchildrens). https://www.ucsfbenioffchildrens.org/conditions/obes ity/#:~:text=A%20child%20with%20one%20obese,gai n%20varies%20for%20different%20people.

WebMD. (n.d.). *High calorie foods*. Nourish. https://www.webmd.com/diet/high-calorie-foods#1

Yau, Y. H., & Potenza, M. N. (2013). Stress and eating behaviors. *Minerva Endocrinologica, 38*(3), 255–267. https://www.ncbi.nlm.nih.gov/pmc/articles/PMC4214 609/